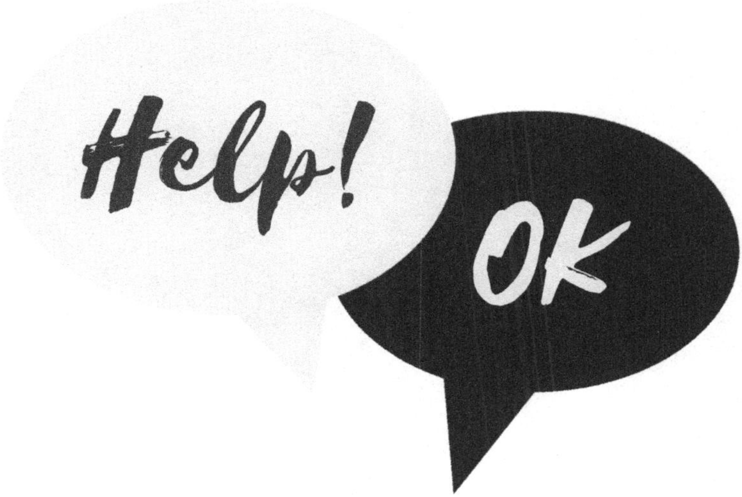
Help!
OK

Help! OK

When "Help!" Meets an "OK" *Magic* Can Happen

RICHARD O. MORGAN

with STEVE HALL

Cookies and Oxygen

PUBLISHING

Cookies and Oxygen Publishing
www.cookiesandoxygen.co.uk

Originally Published in 2015 by Self Published as *Help! Ok. Therapy (sans) Therapists*

Fully Revised and Updated Version First Published in Great Britain in 2018
by Cookies and Oxygen Publishing

ISBN
978-1-912403-05-9 (Paperback)
978-1-912403-04-2 (Ebook)

Printed and bound by Kindle Direct Publishing

02

This book was typeset in Adobe Caslon Pro, Selima, Steelfish, and Guardian Sans Condensed.

Cover design by Steve Hall

AUTHOR'S NOTE

In 2017 I had a collection of fascinating case histories which I had put into writing under a common theme: not only are relationships essential for a balanced life, they can be powerfully therapeutic.

A fairly scrappy collection—that is all they were until I made contact with Steve Hall.

Steve took my writings and skilfully turned them into a book. He took the rough ore of my thoughts and experiences and put them through the refiner's fire of his editorial skills to extract the pure verbal gold that is presented in *Help! OK*.

Whenever the first person is used, it refers to me. In the cases I relate, obviously I have changed all the names. Real names have been changed in a way which hopefully reflects where I met each client—the UK or France.

Richard O. Morgan

June 2018

To Frances Janusz, who has accompanied me on every step along the journey which led to this book. To my every "Help!" she has always replied, "OK."

CONTENTS

CHAPTER 1

A Mother's Kiss

Gotcha! thought Dawn. Her hypnotherapist had just asked her to undress down to her underwear and lie on a table for a massage. Little did he know she was a journalist posing as a patient. A hypnotherapist who asked his female patients to remove their clothes would make for a great lead story in an exposé of fake therapists.

It all started when I got a phone call from my friend Dave. He was a jovial freelance reporter who specialised in scruple-free journalism, selling mostly to rags like *The News of the World* and the *Sunday People*. It was the late 1970s and treating all kinds of ailments and afflictions by hypnosis was becoming increasingly popular.

"Could you give me a hand in weeding out suspicious-looking hypnotherapists?" he asked me. Anybody could claim to be a hypnotherapist without any training or qualifications—they still can—so there will always be a fair number who are only offering their services in order to take advantage of other's vulnerability.

Dave figured, since I was a hypnotherapist myself, I'd know not only the right questions a prospective patient would ask but also how to spot a phoney. "If you come across any who sound weird to you, just give me their names, and we'll take it from there."

I sat down with a pile of Yellow Pages and spent several days calling hypnotherapists in England and Wales—ignoring those in Scotland or Northern Ireland to limit travel expenses. Most of the people I spoke to were warm and friendly and wouldn't be drawn in by my excessive curiosity. However, I managed to compile a list of around thirty hypnotherapists I felt might be worth taking a closer look at. Some of them were very weird indeed. At the top of my list was a man who told me that not only did he have "special powers" of hypnosis, but he also had been initiated in oriental techniques of massage for patients who were too tense to be put into a trance. I was not surprised when Dave gave this therapist's name to a young, attractive freelance reporter who, like himself, didn't complicate her work with scruples.

Dawn made an appointment, and I gave her a short briefing. I suggested that she appear nervous, which would allow our potential groper to suggest a massage. She was a black belt in Judo, so she didn't fear for her safety. She also decided to present a genuine health problem that had bothered her for a couple of years—a mysterious back ache, which her doctor thought was linked to her life style of burning the candle at both ends.

When Dawn turned up for her appointment, she was amused to see our man wearing a white coat to make himself look serious and "medical." After ten minutes, he invited her to remove her clothes and he set about "massaging" her. There was no particularly intimate contact or flagrant groping, but Dawn felt he was getting an unnecessary "eye-full," Benny Hill style.

He suggested Dawn would need ten more sessions after which her back pains would be completely cured. She promised to go away, think about it, and call him back to fix further appointments.

Later, as Dawn wrote up her story, Dave prepared to deliver the *coup de grâce*. The following morning, he went to the hypnotherapist's home, accompanied by a photographer. There were the usual protestations, "I've helped hundreds of people... I have a real gift... This is going to ruin me." All to no avail, of course. All of this was duly photographed and noted.

This story, and several others, was published the following Sunday. Unsurprisingly, when Dave called for a follow-up comment, our man had disappeared.

However, the most fascinating detail never made it into a newspaper. Dawn told us her back pains had disappeared after her phoney consultation. Weeks later, she was still pain-free.

So, what was going on?

~

Serge left prison after serving eight years of a thirteen-year sentence. He had been planning to live off of a little stash of gold he had entrusted to his mother before going down. Unfortunately, his mother had gradually sold the gold over the years and spent the proceeds—mostly in a Casino in Monte Carlo.

While in prison, Serge had obtained O-levels, A-levels, and a degree in sociology. This sounds impressive until you factor in how his sentence would be reduced by one year for every educational certificate he obtained. Let's just say he wasn't motivated by a desire to better himself. However, like many former inmates, there was little he could add to his CV that would tempt somebody to employ him. How was he going to earn a living?

When I met Serge fours years later, he was living in the lap of luxury just outside Toulouse, France. As it turns out that would not last very long, but one sunny day as we sipped cocktails under a parasol beside his swimming pool, Serge told me his story.

A couple of days after his release, for want of anything better to do, he had picked up the free ads paper to look through the job offers. Finding nothing, he continued reading the next rubric "Business Opportunities." Nothing there either, but then he saw the heading "Sciences Ésotériques." Intrigued, he read through promise after promise made by astrologers, fortune-tellers, magicians, healers, and an astonishing number of marabous. (A marabou, by the way, is usually of North African origin and is a cross between a holy man who uses the Quran and a snake-oil salesman.) It occurred to Serge he had found the ideal solution to his vocation problem. No employer, no CV's, no training, and no experience was required.

Serge decided to become a Master of the Occult Sciences.

A week later, Serge had rented a grubby little office and installed a desk and two chairs. For himself, there was an imposing, leather, executive office chair, while his client's seat was a humble, plastic school chair.

He had noticed that the marabous in the ads had called themselves either "Docteur" or "Maître" (Master), rather than the less impressive Monsieur (Mister). So, he decided to call himself Maître Serge La Vie. He paid for a series of small ads, opting for a simple message: "Master Serge La Vie—all problems solved—love, health, work. Money-back guarantee."

He chose a pragmatic, uncomplicated approach to meeting with a client. He would sit opposite them, arms crossed over his wide chest, fix them with his dark, fierce eyes and ask, "What is your problem?" He would listen in complete silence until the client had finished. Then he would say, "I will take care of that. Two hundred francs."

And that was it.

Of course, this was a con. Serge did absolutely nothing to take care of his client's problems.

Within a couple of months his appointments diary was full. His fees varied according to how far Serge felt he could push his luck. He was able to move into a posher office and, after only a year, buy a nice house with the aforementioned swimming pool.

Most of his clients were not only satisfied with him, they recommended him to their friends.

The examples abound but the one concerning a Toulouse pharmacist is typical. The unfortunate man was convinced his house was haunted. Unexplained noises, objects which moved on their own, power cuts, not to mention the "bad luck" which had beset him and his family since moving into this house.

Serge listened in silence as usual.

"I will take care of that. Ten thousand francs in cash. On my desk."

The pharmacist asked Serge to wait for half an hour while he went to the bank to withdraw the cash. On his return, he offered the wad of bank notes to Serge, who told him, "I said on my desk." The twenty 500-franc notes were timidly placed on the desk and the pharmacist left without any further comment from Serge.

Not even a "thank you." In fact, certainly not a "thank you." Just his usual awe-inducing silence.

A week later, Serge received an excited phone call: "Thank you, Master, all the manifestations have stopped. My family and I are so grateful to you. We can start to live again. Oh, and you'll be getting a call from my father-in-law. He desperately needs your help."

Serge was very creative in his approach to "taking care" of people's problems. He started offering to perform special ceremonies the night of the Full Moon. Obviously, these were very expensive fake ceremonies. The only drawback was that they could only be proposed once a month, so he invented another ceremony that could be performed the night of the New Moon too. He then came up with the idea to tell his clients that these ceremonies were performed by a group of people all initiated in the Dark Arts. Each of these people needed paying and Serge's income took a sharp up-turn.

The money kept rolling in because his clients kept on being satisfied with the results.

Alas, Serge was to spend another short spell in prison. But this time it was not for armed robbery or drug dealing. He lost a fight with the tax man.

Soon after his second release from prison, Serge entered my flat without knocking and made his way to the kitchen to get the cafetière working. He called through to me, "Do you know what your Path of Life is?"

"I beg your pardon?"

He appeared at the door, holding a packet of ground coffee, "You heard me. Do you know what your Path of Life is?"

"Er, I don't think so...."

"So how do you know if you're realising your full potential if you don't know what you're meant to do with your life?"

He was grinning his mischievous grin by now. I feared the worst.

"OK. What have you found now to separate people from their money?"

"No, seriously," (with Serge this usually meant the opposite). "I've been reading up about numerology. It's brilliant! Everything in your life is determined by numbers—"

I cut him off and said, "Go and get the coffee, come and sit down and tell me all about it."

He was so excited he couldn't sit still. He kept standing up and sitting down again, waving his arms around, and spilling his coffee. "I've just read a brilliant book by an American, Kevin Quinn Avery. It's called *The Numbers of Life: The Hidden Power in Numerology*. Numbers have vibrations which act upon you from the moment you are born. Your date of birth is numbers, right? And every letter in the alphabet has a hidden number. That means if you know somebody's full name and their date of birth you can tell them what their Path of Life is."

"And...."

"You can see their past, present, and future."

He could see I was sceptical.

"Let's do an experiment," he continued, "Give me the name and date of birth of someone you know in the UK. I'll draw up their numerology chart and tell you stuff about them that will amaze you."

Pouring a second cup of coffee, I decided to play the game, and gave him the information he would need in order to amaze me. Obviously, it concerned somebody about whom he knew nothing.

After a few minutes he had covered four sheets of paper with numbers, columns, geometrical shapes, and diagrams. It looked very impressive. Ten minutes later he announced, "That's all I've learned to do so far. Are you ready?"

"Go ahead," I replied a little nervously.

As I had imagined, he started with lots of generalisations which could have applied to just about anybody. Then he said, "In 1976 there was a divorce."

I sat up in surprise. "Well, yes, actually—"

"I'm not asking you, I'm telling you. Just shut up and listen."

He continued, "There were two children. They changed countries in 1980 or 1981...." Indeed, it was astonishing. Whenever he ventured outside of his fuzzy generalisations, he described the reality as I knew it.

Serge explained that in order to draw up a numerology chart, all numbers had to be reduced to a single figure between 1 and 9. Since I was born on 17th August 1946, my Path of Life could be determined by simple additions, until we got down to one number. He added all the numbers in my date of birth together: 1 + 7 + 8 + 1 + 9 + 4 + 6 = 36. Then, to get the required single figure, he separated 36 into its constituent digits: 3 + 6 = 9.

Just as an astrologist would tell me I am a Leo, a numerologist would tell me I am a "9." The "vibrations" of the number 9 have been acting upon me from the moment I was born. They will influence me throughout my entire life, prodding me to go in the right direction in order to fulfil my destiny. Whenever things go seriously wrong in a person's life, it is because they have strayed from their Path of Life vibrations. Serge told me that as a "9":

> "You have great compassion and idealism. It is in giving that you find satisfaction. You have a broad outlook on life. You tend to see the big picture rather than the minute details. You are rarely prejudiced and you accept the social biases of other people. You are a true egalitarian. You are also imaginative and creative. Because of your strong social consciousness, you could be an effective politician, lawyer, judge, minister, teacher, or healer. Vocations that require self-sacrifice and have a clear social impact are common among nines."

Even though he was obviously only repeating something he had memorised, as a former teacher, and currently a practising hypnotherapist I thought, *what's not to like in that?*

"So, what about the name, and the hidden numbers behind the letters?" I asked him.

He showed me a little diagram:

1	2	3	4	5	6	7	8	9
A	B	C	D	E	F	G	H	I
J	K	L	M	N	O	P	Q	R
S	T	U	V	W	X	Y	Z	

Then he laboriously wrote down the number values for Richard Oliver Morgan. A swift addition to reduce everything to a number between 1 and 9, first the vowels, then the consonants, then all the letters. Using just these three numbers, he "described" my personality, strengths, and weaknesses, and all the rest.

	9			1			6		9		5			6			1		= 37 = 10 = 1
R	I	C	H	A	R	D	O	L	I	V	E	R	M	O	R	G	A	N	
9		3	8		9	4		3		4		9	4		9	7		5	= 74 = 11 = 2
																			= 3

The "1" extracted from the vowel values reveals my "Soul Urge."

The "2" extracted from the consonant values reveals my "Realisation."

And, as you have already guessed, the "3" from the addition of my vowel and consonant values is the "Expression of my Personality."

I detected a lot of truth in Serge's explanations. Naturally, I started studying numerology myself, interested to see how it could help my patients or better equip me to help them.

~

Fast forward two years.

While I was visiting a friend in London, she told me that she had a friend who was looking for a reliable numerologist. (Don't laugh at the oxymoron!) Would I be interested in giving him a consultation?

The friend in question was a Harley Street osteopath on the point of going bankrupt after a vicious and expensive divorce. Apparently, his wife had not taken kindly to his having a mistress.

I went to his posh, Harley Street office, armed with my charts and numbers and calculations. Knowing that he was experiencing financial difficulties, I told him he didn't need to pay me immediately. If, at some later date, he felt my interpretation of his numbers had been helpful, he could send me a cheque when he was in a position to do so.

After listening to an account of his current woes, including the threat of bankruptcy and psoriasis, I launched into my reading. To say he was impressed would be an understatement. Two months later I received a cheque in the post, accompanied by an embarrassingly grateful letter.

However, there was a problem. For me, not my Harley Street client. Back in France, I was looking over his chart when I spotted I had made a simple mistake in my additions right at the very beginning. This meant everything that was based upon these numbers was numerologically wrong.

I remembered how he had nodded his head in enthusiastic agreement as I gave details of his past and present life. Since I am basically honest, I described his personality as revealed by the numbers not sparing him anything. He got the lot—the good, the bad, the ugly... and worse. He admitted it was all true.

But I had been using the wrong numbers!

Since this doctor's life had considerably improved since the day we met, I chose not to enlighten him about my error.

~

You may be tempted to dismiss these stories as coincidences or happy accidents. However, if Serge was successful, it was because his clients were satisfied to the point of recommending him to other people. After the first few months he no longer needed to pay for advertising. People went to him with a problem, Serge "took care it," and their problem disappeared. With so many success stories keeping him in business, a coincidence stops being a coincidence and turns into a pattern. But how and why?

Was Serge employing the power of suggestion to exploit human gullibility? Almost certainly. But when Serge typically said no more than three short, blunt sentences to his client, where does this suggestion get its power?

And what about Dawn's cure? Not only was she sceptical, she was in a consulting room with the intention of exposing the therapist as a con artist and a pervert. A situation in which she would be totally resistant to any form of suggestion... wouldn't she?

And my Numerology reading based on all the wrong numbers? It shouldn't have worked, yet for my client there was an extremely positive outcome. Heck, he even paid me.

In spite of a therapist's approach or motive or mistakes, all therapy meets with a certain degree of success. Which got me thinking about what these stories have in common:

- There is a person with a problem.
- The problem is expressed verbally to somebody who is listening.
- The problem is heard by someone claiming to be able to help.
- Whether that claim is believed seems to be irrelevant.
- Whether that claim is true seems to be equally irrelevant.
- The person's problem is no longer an issue.

A mother of a small child who has just hurt herself, may say to her, "Let mummy kiss it better." This is not a true claim. Kisses do not heal wounds. However, they can reduce the suffering caused by physical pain.

Were Serge's words, "I will take care of that," a sort of verbal motherly kiss?

Was Dawn's choice to speak about a real problem—when she could have invented one—an involuntary child-like cry for help?

What was happening in the osteopath's Harley Street office that led to a wrong numerology reading being so healing?

Even though it was involuntary, Dawn, the pharmacist, and the osteopath all entered into a mother-child relationship with their therapist by saying, "Help me."

Do all therapies meet with some success because they are all variations of a mother's kiss? I would later discover I was on the right track.

CHAPTER 2

I Wasn't Expecting That

Have you ever said, "My mind just went completely blank"? Perhaps when failing to recall someone's name or when you cannot remember where you left your house key. We obviously do not mean our mind has gone completely blank—fortunately, that only occurs in death—instead we mean our brain momentarily stopped working in the way we expected it to. We experienced a temporary disruption to our usual mental processes. Brain freeze. Cognitive dissonance. Mind blank.

Hypnotists seek to duplicate this brief state of mental disconnection. Their aim is to by-pass the analytical part of our mind. One of the most common techniques they use to switch off our critical thinking is called the pattern interrupt.

I found this example of the handshake interrupt via Google:

> When greeting somebody you hold out your hand as if to shake their hand.

> Anticipating that you will immediately shake their hand, they automatically extend their right hand to grasp yours.
>
> Before the hands touch, however, you grasp their extended wrist with the thumb and middle finger, raise their arm and at the same time turn the palm of their hand towards their face.
>
> As they stare at their hand you say, "Look at your hand."
>
> At the same time as you do that you move their hand towards their face and say, "Notice the gradually changing focus of your eyes."
>
> When done smoothly and swiftly it immediately puts the recipient into an altered state for a few seconds and allows you to slip in your hypnotic message.

When the brain recognises a pattern, one of the things it does is automatically make predictions as to what will happen next. Reflexes then spontaneously kick in. If an object is thrown towards my head, I duck. If I jump into water, I hold my breath. If a hand is held out to me, I reach out to grab it. When something unexpected happens instead, the pattern is interrupted and our minds lose their predictive capabilities. Our critical faculties momentarily freeze. When healthy scepticism is briefly put on hold, our brain treats any messages we receive as fact. A skilled hypnotist can then sneak in information or instruction without our brains filtering this message.

Shock produces a similar mind blank response. This is why bank robbers and hijackers act rapidly and shout a lot. People become docile as their minds struggle with the out of the ordinary. This reduces the risk of immediate resistance.

In other words, when you find yourself in a surprise situation and you don't know what to do, you will probably do what you are told.

Milton Erickson, the iconic figure of clinical hypnosis in the latter part of the 20th century, is popularly attributed as saying that hypnotherapy is often established "by the utilisation of silly, absurd, irrational, and contradictory statements."

For example, what happens when you reflect upon the absurd question of "*What is the sound of one hand clapping?*"

If you force yourself to form a concept of "clapping"—an action performed with two hands—while only using "one hand," you will immediately run up against cognitive conflict. You might even mentally switch off. Your mind may go blank for a while before sending you running to get a cup of coffee.

The absurd, the irrational, and the contradictory can all produce pattern interrupt.

Are they koans?

> koan / noun
>
> a paradoxical anecdote or riddle without a solution, used in Zen Buddhism to demonstrate the inadequacy of logical reasoning and provoke enlightenment. [1]

Can "blank minds" lead to enlightenment?

An old Moroccan friend once made an interesting observation about Islam. As a practising Muslim there was no mockery in his words, just a sparkle in his wise old eyes. "Islam both allows and forbids polygamy," he said. "Allah allows a man to have four wives.

But then He seems to render it impossible by commanding that all four wives be treated equally."

Contradiction?

The Christian gospel is full of exhortations to be righteous. Why, then, do we read in Romans 3:10, "There is none righteous, no, not one."

Impossible paradox?

Usually, when we are confronted with paradoxes or contradictions, our critical faculties—silently guided by our world view and steered by confirmation biases—will enable us to either resolve the paradox, explain it away, or just abandon it as meaningless nonsense.

However, there is an alternative which involves neither explaining nor rejecting. It has been called the "willing suspension of disbelief."

Or blind faith.

Or passionate love.

Or the maternal instinct.

Or feminine intuition.

In his book, *Why People Believe Weird Things,* Michael Shermer claims that:

> Rarely do any of us sit down before a table of facts, weigh them pro and con, and choose the most logical and rational belief, regardless of what we previously believed. Instead, the facts of the world come to us

> through the coloured filters of the theories, hypotheses, hunches, biases, and prejudices we have accumulated through our lifetime. We then sort through the body of data and select those most confirming what we already believe, and ignore or rationalise away those that are disconfirming. [2]

We are not as logical or rational as we would like to believe. Most of the time we do not employ our critical faculties to analyse what is going on. For example, you never hear anyone say, "Our eyes met across the crowded room, and I knew I had to have a background check done on him." Or, "I will love you forever and ever and ever... unless due diligence turns up something I'm not happy with."

Horse breeders are very choosy about the pedigrees of the animals that they put together for a romp in the hay. Humans less so, apparently. The divorce courts are full of people perhaps wishing they had been a bit more objective in their choices, but *"C'est la vie."*

Isn't it?

~

A type of pattern interrupt is often expressed by the words, "This is the first time I've ever told anyone about this." In those words, there is a tacit message, "You can do what you want with me now." This state of mind is transitory (fortunately!) but whatever the therapist says or does will be accepted in a non-critical way—foot massage, healing hands on the head, magic incantations.

When we open up for the first time in our lives, we become vulnerable for a short while.

The most beneficial and non-invasive thing a therapist can do is... just listen. When he shows his patient they have his undivided attention, he is sending them a powerful message:

- I am interested in what you have to say.
- You are making sense to me, so I understand.
- I will not judge and reject you.
- Everything you say will be taken seriously.
- At this moment you are important to me.
- In my eyes, you can exist as you really are—no need for the masks of social behaviour.

The patient consequently has some or all of the following reactions:

- Wow, somebody is interested in what I have to say.
- I really think I'm being understood at last.
- This is so weird—I'm not being rejected or judged.
- I'm being taken seriously. Isn't this too good to be true?
- I really have the feeling that I'm important to this person.
- At last, I can just be myself. What an incredible relief.

Having someone listen to their problem, can be sufficient for a person to feel better. It will cause them to start delving into their own resources to find a solution from within themselves of which they were previously unaware.

This therapeutic context, in whatever form, contains the elements of *contradiction*. The patient experiences *surprise*—this has never happened to me before—and *pattern interrupt*—this is so different from what goes on in "normal" life.

I have a friend who is a psychiatrist and psychotherapist. He once told me that one of the most powerful things he had ever said to a patient was, "Hi."

After pouring out her woes in words and tears, his patient lapsed into an inevitable helpless silence. She eventually wiped her eyes and looked at my friend. He just looked back, and said, "Hi."

With that one word, his patient felt, for the first time, that she existed in her own right. All because her existence had been acknowledged.

But, hang on a sec—did my friend need his years of study, and his wall full of framed diplomas in order to say, "Hi"?

Or is it a case of the plumber's bill?

A woman calls in a plumber when her washing machine breaks down. The plumber arrives, studies the machine, then produces a hammer and gives it a hefty whack.

The washing machine starts working again, and the plumber presents a bill for $200.

"Two hundred dollars?" says the woman. "All you did was hit it with the hammer."

So, the plumber gives her an itemised bill—Hitting washing machine with a hammer: $5. Knowing where to hit it: $195.

You will be able to decide for yourself later. Maybe.

CHAPTER 3

Jamel and Spinoza

"How much did you pay for that?" asked Jamel, nodding towards my shiny, new briefcase.

While twenty-seven other pupils fought over the choice of places on this first day of the new school year, Jamel got straight down to business. Even though this was my first encounter with him, 13-year-old Jamel's reputation had preceded him. The teachers who knew him were unanimous in their advice: "Never buy anything from Jamel, and just let him sleep if you want to get on with your lesson."

Unsure about how to react, I stared severely at his back-to-front baseball cap, which he had failed to remove as per school rule "14(b) Attire." With a languid gesture, he removed his cap. Tending it to me, he said, "If you like it, it's yours for ten francs. And I can get you a briefcase just like yours for thirty francs. Or you can have two for fifty."

Six months later, having bought nothing from Jamel and having allowed him to sleep at the back of the class, I decided it was time to lie to him.

Bottom of the class since the age of eight, Jamel was, in fact, a fairly intelligent child. Very street-wise, certainly. He had a reputation for being a talented rapper and a star on the basketball court. But school was not his thing. I had learned that he often needed to sleep in class because he rarely got to bed early. He was the look-out for his older brother and his friends, who did their nightly business at the foot of a tower block in a largely Arab neighbourhood in Toulouse. He had shared with me that he was thinking of going into contraband cigarettes when he left school since the cost of smoking was increasing every year. Either that or try to make it as a rapper, at which he was quite talented.

As a teacher, I was not in the habit of lying to my pupils. However, on occasion I had lied to a perennially underachieving student with the aim of building their self-esteem. These manipulative lies had been effective, so I felt the time was ripe to use one on Jamel. Maybe give him the chance to get something positive out of his schooling.

In the French educational system, tests and exams are marked out of twenty. Many pupils spent their time crossing their fingers to score at least ten—the average. That way, the worst that could be said about them on their term reports was: "Could do better." Across all the subjects, Jamel regularly attained an average of 3/20. His average was pushed up to 3 by his performances on the basketball court. His sports teacher loved him. Most teachers had given up on him, accepting that he was just biding his time until he could legally leave school and set up his own business.

It was just before the Easter Holidays in March. The last test of the term. As I returned the papers to anxious pupils, I deliberately held back Jamel's to the end. I gave it to him as his classmates filed out of the room. As usual, I should have given him a symbolic 1/20, but I lied and gave him 4/20 instead—a massive improvement on previous results.

I handed him the paper, and before he had the chance to screw it into a ball and slam-dunk it into the bin, I said, "Well done, Jamel. Four out of twenty. Looks like you might have a talent for English. Maybe it's all that American rap you listen to. Let's see what you can do next term, OK?"

I didn't wait for a reaction. You don't get into discussions with Jamel if you want to avoid everything going pear-shaped.

Why give him 4/20, when the only thing correct in his test was his name? I safely assumed that he had not read Spinoza's brilliant insight in the seventeenth century, when he observed:

> Mere comprehension of a statement entails the tacit acceptance of its being true, whereas disbelief requires a subsequent process of rejection. [3]

Hearing me pronounce the words "four out of twenty," linked to a brief compliment plus a brief explanation (American Rap) forced him to deal with a brand-new concept. In school, he could be worth more than 0/20.

Jamel had long accepted that bottom of the class was his natural place. He had developed standard ways to avoid shame, humiliation, or failure by putting on an air of not caring, ignoring exhortations to "work harder," and over-compensating in other areas. In Jamel's case, he had a good business sense, a great sales spiel, and he gained respect from his peers on the basketball court and through rapping in the playground. He was also very big for his age, which obviously helped too.

But what if school could be something other than a nuisance to be put up with until the age of sixteen? What if an education could give him a chance of accessing a safer form of success?

I exploited the fact he liked me to slip an idea into his mind that he could be worth more than a zero in school. Maybe that would open up new possibilities for Jamel.

Three months later, I overheard a couple of teachers in the staff-room discussing Jamel. They were saying things like, "I don't know what's happened to him, but he's starting to get some good results in Maths," and "Yes, I've noticed that he often wakes up in Life Sciences."

Something seemed to have changed. I was transferred to a different school at the end of that year and I lost sight of Jamel.

~

In his paper, *Functional Neuroimaging of Belief, Disbelief, and Uncertainty*, Sam Harris, ever the pragmatist, reports:

> Several psychological studies appear to support Spinoza's conjecture that the mere comprehension of a statement entails the tacit acceptance of its being true, whereas disbelief requires a subsequent process of rejection. Understanding a proposition may be analogous to perceiving an object in physical space: We seem to accept appearances as reality until they prove otherwise. Our behavioural data support this

> hypothesis, in so far as subjects judged statements to be "true" more quickly than they judged them to be "false" or "undecidable." [4]

Unless we have some prior knowledge or experience that immediately contradicts what we've been told, we take things at face-value. We assume a statement is true because to reject it would require extra thought and perhaps even some research. We are therefore hesitant to judge something as untrue.

Jamel—and he was not the only example during my time as a teacher—heard a compliment from me which he should have rejected as false. It contradicted everything other teachers had been telling him for years. Had he read Spinoza or Sam Harris, the logical thing for Jamel to have done would have been to look at his test to see how he had managed to score four points. It did not occur to him to do this. Had the numbers 4 and 20 been related to the price of dubiously acquired briefcases, Jamel would have been a little more analytical. But this was not the case.

Of course, context is everything. I had established a positive relationship with Jamel. He liked me. He would have liked to have given me the pleasure of seeing him obtain better results in English even though I never insisted or chided him to do this. On a couple of occasions, I had even recorded a couple of "mixes" for Jamel to use when rapping. I was therefore credible in his eyes.

Why would I cease to be credible when I said, "Well done"?

Had Jamel not trusted me, my words would have fallen on deaf ears. However, he did trust me. So instead of seeking information to verify or invalidate the information I had given him, he unwittingly found himself in a dilemma: what do I do with this?

My dual lie—the marks I gave him and my compliment—were initially accepted as true. They were neither examined nor rejected, meaning they bypassed Jamel's intellectual faculties and accepted as fact. *Four out of twenty. A talent for English. What could next term hold?* My encouragement made him feel good. He experienced a positive mental sensation.

Is this a case where it can be advantageous to believe a lie and act on it as if it were a truth? Where accepting false information actually provokes a positive change in attitude and behaviour, such that the lie is no longer a lie, *per se*? Rather, does it become a self-fulfilling prophecy?

The neuroscientist Robert Burton has pointed out:

> [Modern biology] is telling us that despite how certainty feels, it is neither a conscious choice nor even a thought process. Certainty and similar states of "knowing what we know" arise out of primary brain mechanisms that, like love or anger, function independently of rationality or reason. Feeling correct or certain isn't a deliberate conclusion or conscious choice. It is a mental sensation that happens to us. [5]

"Whether you think you can or whether you think you can't, you're right!" are words often attributed to Henry Ford. They are usually presented as a remedy for overcoming failure and moving towards success. The false implication is that all you need to do is change what you believe about yourself. However, it fails to take into account how we do not get to create our own self-image. We will always tend to see ourselves as others have seen us—starting, of course, with mummy and maybe daddy. After the first few years of life, our performances in the real world will be an expression of our genuine capabilities issuing from, and sometimes in conflict with, our beliefs about ourselves.

In adult life it becomes very difficult to change our beliefs about ourselves. Eight years of psychoanalysis? Maybe. Brain injury? Possibly. Being loved and accepted? Probably, though there is no guarantee. A life-induced catharsis? Perhaps. Can these changes be self-induced? Certainly not.

Conditioned thought patterns or reflexes are very tenacious, and notoriously difficult to modify or remove. However, a "dramatic shock" can often do the trick.

The best example of being shocked into change is the story of Pavlov's dogs. Many of you will know Pavlov conditioned his dogs to drool at the sound of a bell, but few know about what happened to his dogs in his laboratory in 1924.

On 22nd September 1924, Pavlov's laboratories in Leningrad were flooded. His dogs were forced to swim to the top of their low cages to avoid being drowned. Pavlov's assistants managed to unlock the cages and force the panicking dogs under the water in order to escape through the now open doors.

All the conditioned dogs were saved, however, there were some exceptional consequences. In some of them the conditioned reflexes had disappeared as if they had never been formed.

William Sargant—notorious for his over-enthusiastic belief in the effectiveness of pre-frontal lobotomies—was perhaps the first to suggest that a similar "dramatic shock" was responsible for the apparent character changes observed in many cases of religious conversion. He suspected that something was going on in the brain. [6]

When the mind is confronted with new information in a way that bypasses the critical faculties, it has to come up with a new mental framework to house it in. This new structure will almost certainly entail a change in belief and/or attitude. We do not change our fundamental beliefs by simply telling ourselves, "I am going to stop believing x and start believing y." Instead, we require outside input for our mindset to alter.

Change requires an external factor. Something that interrupts the current pattern of our lives and suggests a better way to live. It's unsurprising how often change occurs when a demand for help meets an offer of help. However, Jamel's story is an example of change being induced in the absence of any plea for aid. Some people no longer believe there is a solution to their suffering or they believe that their problem will disappear with the passage of time. Therefore, they do not ask for help. Often the worst thing we can do for these people is to ask them if they want help. Their reactions can be very violent. Nevertheless, there are still ways we can interact with people who could benefit from assistance, where we don't position ourselves as the "helper." My approach with Jamel demonstrates one such way.

Generally, four elements can be identified:

- A source of pain, suffering, or stress.
- An apparent impossibility of internal changes occurring to alleviate or remove the problem.
- An external intervention which creates an entirely new form of cognitive dissonance.
- The emergence of a new attitude and/or behaviour which reduces the pain, suffering, or stress.

~

I saw Jamel again thirteen years later. I was waiting in line at a checkout in my local supermarket when I was shaken out of my reverie by a vigorous tap on the shoulder. Startled, I turned around and saw a tall, beaming young man.

"Mr Morgan! Do you remember me? Jamel? You were my English teacher in 7th grade!"

"How could I forget you, Jamel? How are you keeping? You look well."

"I didn't go into cigarettes after all. I work in computer sales now. I got a HND from the technical college. I'm married and we've got two children."

"And your family, your brothers, and sisters?"

His face clouded over. "I'm afraid Hakim is still in prison. He got five years for drug dealing and possession of a firearm. He should be getting out in a few months."

Did my "lie" thirteen years previously help Jamel avoid a similar fate? I suppose we'll never know for sure.

But I know what I like to think....

CHAPTER 4

Hypnotherapy

When inducing a trance state, the traditional hypnotherapist doesn't say to his patient, "We're going to have a nice chat." (That would come later with fitted kitchen salesmen and Neuro-Linguistic Programming). He instead invites the subject to listen in silence and obey. And at £85 per session, one tends to be positively inclined to shut up and do what you're told.

By using specific verbal methods, the hypnotherapist associates his words with sensations the subject will genuinely experience. During the session, at least, the subject will therefore attribute special powers to him. However, the therapist has none. What is actually happening is that a regressive relationship is being established. A reversion to a mother-child relationship is taking place.

In a relationship where one person plays a parental role (almost a uniquely maternal one), the other person will, depending on the context, regress to childlike behaviour. In hypnotherapy, the therapist assumes this maternal mantle to enable their client to abandon normal "adult" behaviour momentarily. On the therapist's couch, the magic of the baby and her mother is re-awakened. Mummy partially helped us to become what we are as adults. A new, temporary Mummy can plug into the vulnerability and unquestioning trust we had as a child, in order to help modify or "heal" certain parts of the adult personality.

And it often works.

Don't ask me how I know.

A common misperception about hypnotherapy is that if the hypnotherapist uses a calm, soothing tone of voice, then he is reproducing a mother image. If he uses an authoritarian order-giving voice, then he is playing the role of the father. This is unlikely. In my experience, the authoritarian order-barking type of trance induction is only used by stage hypnotists. This places the subjects—who are also intimidated by the spotlights and the audience—in a similar situation to passengers in a plane that is being hi-jacked. For a brief period, the subject is unable to think clearly and rationally.

In a therapeutic situation, not only does the hypnotist become "Mummy," he is reconstructing through his words the dynamics of a relationship that was formed during the very earliest stage of the child's life. This bond was originally formed during the nine months they spent in their mother's womb. It is then cemented during a baby's early months or years, where almost without exception the mother is the child's primary care-give.

In western societies, the father has at best been a secondary influence during a child's formative years. Psychoanalysts and ethologists have shown us that the father, or the father figure, is designated by the mother. Before the appearance of DNA testing, only the mother could be absolutely sure she was the mother. The father and child had to take the mother's word for it when one man was designated "father."

A human being therefore carries a maternal imprint thought their entire life. When this relational phenomenon is recreated in adult life through the words spoken to us on the hypnotherapist's couch, there is something in the limbic system of our brains which causes us to switch to this regressive state.

We momentarily become a child again.

~

I would occasionally run hypnotherapy courses—usually in response to a demand. Inevitably, in each group, there would be at least one individual who would boastfully and noisily announce something like, "I want to learn how to hypnotise other people, but I know that I could never be hypnotised myself. My personality is too strong."

When the time came to demonstrate a typical trance induction, I would invariably choose this person to be the guinea-pig. I would use what is known as the hidden double bind technique.

Having invited my volunteer to stand beside me in front of the group, I would first ask two other members of the group to stand behind him to catch him when he fell backwards under my "influence." This caused my subject to create useful muscular tensions. He was preparing to resist any inclination to fall backwards, but by bracing himself he was actually reducing his stability. But of course, he didn't know that.

I was setting the scene.

Then I would set the trap during a short, preparatory exchange:

"You believe that your personality is so strong that you could never be hypnotised, right?"

Smiling nervously, "Absolutely."

"I believe you. In fact, I want you to promise to resist everything I am going to say to you. Will you do that?"

Less confidently, because he is becoming suspicious, "Yes."

"OK. Let's begin."

Then I would allow a few seconds of uncomfortable silence. Everybody, including my subject would be wondering what was going to happen next.

Adopting a melodramatic, sepulchral "hypnotist's" voice, I would say: "I know that you are going to resist and reject everything I say to you. I accept that there is no way that I can cast my hypnotic influence on you. Your strong personality makes it impossible for me to cause you to fall backwards against your will. You have no sensation of being light-headed. You feel perfectly solid and stable. You do not need two people standing behind you to catch you in case you fall because you are not going to fall backwards. You can not lose balance or start wobbling. You can not feel any irresistible force pushing you backwards."

Usually at this point, my subject would fall backwards into the hands of the two volunteers standing behind him. There would be gasps of awe from the group. It was only at the end of the training session that I would explain what had been happening. After all, I do not possess any strange gifts or powers.

The "double bind" I used, and which never failed, was contained in the sentence: "I want you to promise to resist everything I am going to say to you." When the subject hears a set of contradictory instructions or orders they are meant to be resisting, they become confused. Their critical faculties are temporarily put on hold and their brain will reach for the easiest solution. The path of least resistance. "There's lots of talk about falling, so let's go with that." This happens virtually instantaneously.

Interestingly, studies have shown that even saying to the subject "I don't want you to go to sleep," will actually induce a sensation of drowsiness. The brain's filter will pick up the word "sleep" first and ignore the rest. In order to follow the instruction, the brain has to imagine "sleep" before being able to process the rest of the sentence. Just try telling someone not to yawn and watch what happens.

Of course, hypnosis has actually begun before the patient even arrives in the therapist's office. She knows she is going to be "hypnotised." She has therefore given her consent to being subjected to whatever she imagines hypnosis to be. There is a willing suspension of disbelief as well as a relaxing of vigilance. The therapist then uses the tried and tested techniques of monotony and repetition to further decrease her natural alertness.
The key factor is the association of the helpless with a helper. The passive with the active. On the therapist's couch there is also the horizontal (the baby) with the vertical (the mother).

~

Let's look at a typical trance induction script, so we can analyse what is going on:

> You are lying here listening to the sound of my voice, perhaps wondering how it is that you are going to go into a trance. As you listen to these words, I would like you to focus your gaze on an imaginary spot on the ceiling. That's good. In a few moments I will begin counting. When I say the number one, I would like you to close your eyes, and then on the number two, slowly open them. Continue to open and close your eyes on alternating numbers in this way until your eyes feel so heavy it would be easier and more comfortable to just let them remain closed. Whether your eyes are closed or open, I would like you to keep your focus on that spot on the ceiling. Do not lower your gaze during the numbers on which your eyes are closed, keep your eyes fixed in the same position and imagine you are still gazing at the spot.

You are lying here listening to the sound of my voice...

Why start by stating the obvious? She knows she's lying there listening to the sound of his voice. It corresponds exactly with what she is experiencing. Therefore, words and sensations are being linked and the therapist's words are beginning to become trustworthy. There is also a subtle association of passivity with activity: "You are lying here listening..." with "the sound of my voice." I'm the one who's doing the talking here. Just shut up and listen.

...perhaps wondering how it is that you are going to go into a trance.

Not *if* you are going to go into a trance. We are both going to assume that it will happen. You may be wondering how—implying "But who cares? I'm in charge here."

As you listen to these words...

Repetition. Always lots of repetition.

Previously, it was "listening to the sound of my voice," now it's "listen to these words." The sound of the therapist's voice is subtly linked to "these words" in general.

Amongst the many functions of the brain, there is one very closely linked to survival. Its task is to recognise any changes to your environment and alert the conscious part of the mind. A classic example is falling asleep in a noisy plane cabin and being awoken by a change in the sound of the engines. Once your brain realised that the annoying noise did not pose any threat to your life, it stopped worrying about it and let you go to sleep. When the noise changed, it woke you up. Familiarity is sleep-inducing. Change sets off alarms.

...I would like you to focus your gaze on an imaginary spot on the ceiling.

The therapist begins to gently impose his will. He does so by requiring the subject to be attentive to internal data sources rather than external realities. The spot isn't really there—it's just imaginary. So, if the subject is to gaze at it, where is she looking?

However, she dutifully looks up at the ceiling. Concentrating one's gaze on a spot or an object which is slightly elevated will cause rapid fatigue in the ocular muscles. There will be a spontaneous need to close the eyes. This is one of the reasons why it is hard to stay awake during long sermons.

That's good...

A reassuring compliment, or as they used to say in Transactional

Analysis, a verbal stroke. For many of us raised in a western country, it will also evoke at some level the words from Genesis: "And God saw that it was good."

In a few moments I will begin counting. When I say the number one, I would like you to close your eyes...

You were wondering how you were going to go into a trance? No problem. Let's start with a very simple, infant-friendly instruction. (Alert level drops a few more degrees.) "All you have to do is close your eyes when you hear the number one. Now who's a clever girl?"

To avoid alerting the brain, the request is expressed in gentle terms, "I would like you to...." Meaning, "If you do that, Mummy is going to be very happy with you."

Then comes the first serious act of manipulation the therapist uses to coax the subject into abandoning vigilance:

And then on the number two, slowly open them...

Have you ever tried opening your eyes slowly? They're either open or closed, aren't they? So, an impossible request sneaks into the monologue. Usually the subject does not detect the impossibility of opening her eyes slowly, so she just lets the word slip by. As she will later let many words slip by and slink into her subconscious to work their magic.

And what a soothing word "slowly" is. The very sound of it is soporific.

Continue to open and close your eyes on alternating numbers in this way until your eyes feel so heavy it would be easier and more comfortable to just let them remain closed.

Repeat one, two, one, two, until you've had enough of it.

Again, repetition. Nothing for the corpus callosum to get excited about. Furthermore, for most first-time subjects, this allays any anxieties that the therapist is going to make her close her eyes against her will. "Look, it's just happening naturally because you are more comfortable that way."

Whether your eyes are closed or open, I would like you to keep your focus on that spot on the ceiling. Do not lower your gaze during the numbers on which your eyes are closed, keep your eyes fixed in the same position and imagine you are still gazing at the spot.

We've got to get your ocular muscles good and tired. So, you just keep on looking at something that isn't there, OK? By being simultaneously soothing and confusing, the therapist lulls the brain's alert mechanisms into a sense of security where they are no longer needed.

After looking upwards for long enough, her eyes will naturally want to remain closed. This is why, in the trance induction, the therapist asks the subject to maintain this tiring eye position, even when the eyes are shut. He also reinforces the sensation of sleepiness by the using keywords, like "trance," "easier," and "more comfortable." In order to not alarm the subject, he usually avoids the word "sleep." He knows full well that closed eyes and sensations of simple comfort are linked with going to sleep in the subject's mind.

Yes, you've got it. Trance induction is a lullaby.

"Go to sleep my baby..." Mummy is taking care of everything.

CHAPTER 5

What's in a Title?

When I was a practising hypnotherapist, the first contact I usually had with a patient was over the phone. Rarely did they ring me and say, "I'm calling to make an appointment," like you would when ringing a doctor or a dentist, though it did happen sometimes. Instead, the caller would mainly ask me questions about hypnotherapy and sometimes, in seeking reassurance, they would ask me what my qualifications were or how much experience I had.

Whenever someone asked me about my qualifications, I always gave them the same answer. Which, while being true, they should have found alarming.

"Excuse my asking, but do you mind telling me what your qualifications are?"

"Sure. I read a book once, a long time ago."

My answer never deterred anyone from coming to see me. Unbelievable but true.

When a person called me, they were already saying "Help!" This is why it was extremely rare for someone to hang up before asking for an appointment. We both knew why they had called. My responsibility was to address that basic plea. Those callers who asked me about my qualifications were really asking whether they could trust me. And we both knew there was no satisfactory answer to that question.

Where my flippant answer should have dissuaded them, it did the opposite. They appreciated that I didn't launch into a long litany of degrees and diplomas. Every caller made an appointment with me after I told them "I read a book once," because nothing else had worked and because they sensed I was going to be real with them.

~

I started practising hypnotherapy in the late 1970s. By then it was widely accepted and was even becoming a respectable way to earn a living. I had previously been a music teacher. I gave that up because of a frustration with my lack of impact within a school setting.

So, I became a hypnotist. Though, not exactly.

I began by reading piles of books about hypnotherapy. I studied Mesmer and Charcot, and from there went on to look at all sorts of altered states of consciousness and how to access them. I read everything I could lay my hands on by Milton Erickson, who specialised in medical hypnosis. I even went as far as plunging into weighty volumes of clinical psychology.

After I had picked up a reasonable knowledge of the theory, I sought out some practical experience. I observed many sessions of hypnotherapy and, of course, was hypnotised myself. One of the people who allowed me to sit in on their appointments was a clinical psychologist who practised hypnotherapy. She soon became a friend. Out of the blue one day, she announced, "I think you could set yourself up as a hypnotherapist now."

I somewhat disingenuously protested that I had no qualifications or diplomas to put on my wall. She didn't see that as an obstacle. Neither did I actually, but I was relying on her to come up with some idea. She told me to create an official-looking certificate which she would sign for me.

A few weeks later, I had rented a small office in the centre of Manchester, furnished it with two chairs, a desk, a couch, and, of course, my fake certificate. The proud final touch was the doorplate: "Richard Morgan – Hypnotherapist."

I put a small ad in some local papers and sat by my phone. My appointments diary filled up very quickly, and I thought, wrongly, that my teaching days were well behind me.

You may think that I am admitting I was a charlatan, a fraud, or a con artist. Well, yes. A bit. In my defence, I will say that I never knowingly made false promises, and I was certainly extremely conscientious and well-intentioned.

~

I have not come across any serious studies that examine people's motives for becoming reflexologists, astrologists, faith healers, channellers, or hypnotherapists. I am personally acquainted with several who privately admit it was an easy way to make money.

Many claim it is a calling or their reason for being on this Earth. "A curious calling" is how Michael Sussman describes the career choice of becoming a psychotherapist. [7]

Freud's daughter, Anna, herself a prominent psychoanalyst, once said, "The most sophisticated defence mechanism I ever encountered was becoming a psychotherapist." [8]

John Fromson, M.D., director of a Massachusetts program for impaired physicians, describes the mental health field as one in which "the odd care for the id." [9]

Regardless of their motive, they all needed a title (official or otherwise) before embarking on a career of helping people. Giving yourself a title such as "Hypnotherapist" or "Psychotherapist" or "Aromatherapist" reassures potential clients and is very good for business. Certainly, for professional purposes, a name-plate saying, "Richard Morgan – A Really Nice Guy" would attract far fewer clients than "Richard Morgan – Hypnotherapist."

A title is also reassuring for the therapist. Not only reassuring but powerfully enabling. It says, "This is not me, Richard Morgan, with all my weaknesses helping you. It is Mr Morgan, the hypnotherapist. I will be doing professional things to you and you will be paying me for my time and expertise." It means the therapist can hide their own insecurities by emphasising how it is the *method* which helps the patient, more than the therapist they are seeing.

Why is such a charade necessary?

What's really in a title?

Having chosen their method (for whatever reason), the therapist can then assume a title. The client is attracted by this title and when she turns up for a consultation, bingo! The therapeutic relationship can begin to take form. Almost without exception, the technique being used is little more than a pretext for creating this relationship. If the approach is not based on manual therapy, the stars, numbers, or plain magic, she will be listened to. If effective listening is taking place, she will also have the feeling of being heard. Maybe for the first time.

Then comes the method, for the patient expects the practitioner to do something to her. The problem here is the patient needs to buy into the model being proposed. If a therapists' method is not accepted as factual, then not only will his patient go elsewhere, he will suffer a puncture in his self-image.

Of course, in most cases, the people seeking help are self-selecting. No one calls a naturopath in order to have her future predicted by the stars. (Maybe they do. Stranger things have been reported...) The patient therefore carries some expectation that the method will help before she even turns up for her appointment. If she finds herself listened to, this method has every chance of being helpful in some way.

Transactional Analysis used to propose an interesting model of the mind. I suppose it still does, but I use the past tense as it was all the rage fifty years ago. It claimed that within all of us there is an Adult, a Parent, and a Child. It will come as no surprise to you that everyone who has undergone this therapy is now walking around with an Adult, a Parent, and a Child inside of them. Does this actually correspond with any objective reality? There is no way of determining this. It could just be a useful model to help patients better understand their own personality. Maybe. It is certainly no worse than the ego, super-ego, and id of the Freudian school of psychoanalysis.

In contrast, the reflexologist will have pretty charts on their walls, showing lines of energy radiating out from every part of the foot to various parts of the body. If, for example, you have a problem with your vocal chords, there is a tiny spot nestling between your big toe and the ball of your foot which needs to be tweaked and massaged. This seems to work for some people.

Cognitive Behavioural Therapy (CBT) is the popular method of the moment. It sounds nice and scientific and appealing, doesn't it? Yet there is nothing new in CBT. Apart from the title.

It's always the title, isn't it?

~

What directs a therapist's choice of method in one direction rather than another? There is not enough research to reach any conclusions. And in fact it probably doesn't matter. There is something much more important going on. The answer lies in something that was often said in France a few years ago, "*Le psychanalyste a remplacé le prêtre.*"

The psychoanalyst has replaced the priest.

In the Roman Catholic sacrament of reconciliation—better known as "confession"—the penitent believes the priest is acting "in persona Christi" (literally "in the person of Christ"), as he speaks the words comprising this sacred rite.

There is a line in the Absolution, used by some priests, which insists on this point:

> My child, (Name), may our Lord and God Christ Jesus
> by the mercy of His love absolve thee from thy sins;

> and I, His unworthy priest, in virtue of the authority committed to me, absolve thee and declare thee absolved of thy sins in the name of the Father, and of the Son, and of the Holy Ghost. Amen. [10]

The priest is saying clearly, "It's not me, it's Christ."

So, what is so special about being a priest? In the Roman Catholic Church, they believe a priest holds authority or power that has been granted by God Himself.

It has not been demonstrated that God or any other super-power has granted therapists any special authority. If you want to see where your therapist's authority comes from, look at the framed certificates hanging on his wall. However, you are unlikely to hear him say, "By the authority vested in me by my CBT certificate, I hereby bring you into the here-and-now." Or if he's a traditionalist, *"...the hic et nunc."*

It might be objected that psychologists, like airplane pilots, need to be highly trained and overseen by some higher authority. Well, yes, sort of.... Though piloting an Airbus 380 and being responsible for the lives of 850 passengers at a time, is a little more pragmatic than tweaking toes or resolving Oedipus complexes.

Just how effective is professional training in producing competent psychotherapists? Alas, many studies and meta-studies (the study of studies) demonstrate it is generally no more effective than simply knowing how to be a reasonably empathetic listener.

> Paraprofessionals achieve clinical outcomes equal to or significantly better than those obtained by professionals. In terms of measurable outcome, professionals may not possess demonstrably superior clinical skills when

> compared with paraprofessionals. Moreover, professional mental health education, training, and experience do not appear to be necessary prerequisites for an effective helping person. [11]

But even paraprofessionals work within a context, which confers a sort of authority.

Who actually needs to be reassured most by the authority of a title? The practitioner or the patient?

Is it possible to find an ordinary friend who can provide a safe place to be heard? Dinah Craik describes such a scenario in her novel from 1859, *A Life for a Life.*

> Thus ended our little talk: yet it left a pleasant impression. True, the subject was strange enough; my sisters might have been shocked at it; and at my freedom in asking and giving opinions. But oh! the blessing it is to have a friend to whom one can speak fearlessly on any subject; with whom one's deepest as well as one's most foolish thoughts come out simply and safely. Oh, the comfort—the inexpressible comfort of feeling safe with a person—having neither to weigh thoughts nor measure words, but pouring them all right out, just as they are, chaff and grain together; certain that a faithful hand will take and sift them, keep what is worth keeping, and then with the breath of kindness blow the rest away.
>
> Somebody must have done a good deal of the winnowing business this afternoon; for in the course of it I gave him as much nonsense as any reasonable man could stand.

If we cannot find a friend to talk to like this, why not?

There is a good answer to this.

CHAPTER 6

Why You Do (or Don't) Need Therapy

Do you feel that you need therapy?

Do you know somebody who, in your opinion, could benefit from counselling?

Before we answer those questions, perhaps we should take a step back and ask, "Who actually needs therapy?"

According to Freud (the legend) everybody should be psychoanalysed. According to some extreme Christians, nobody needs therapy for everyone just needs "saving."

People do not tend to reflect upon what they hope will happen by undertaking therapy. Neither do they reflect upon what they think will happen if they decide not to. Trying to do either is not as simple as it sounds.

When I say, "I need to eat and drink regularly," I know specifically what I need and why I need it. However, when I say "I need therapy," it is not as easy to describe the nature of the thing I need.

Things get more complicated when I ask people, "Why do you think you need therapy?" and "Why do you think your spouse needs therapy?" The answers are rarely the same though one imagines that they should be.

When asked why they need therapy, people will say things like:

"I'm depressed all the time and I don't know what to do to get out of it."

"I feel that there are issues that I need to talk out with somebody."

"I keep getting anxiety attacks that I can't control and I don't know why."

"I have a friend who seems much happier since she went for counselling."

In other words, they will express a problem without spontaneously being able to say why they believe therapy could provide the solution. It is hard to imagine other life situations where this is the case. Usually we know what we need and why we need it. Some needs we can take care of ourselves. Others clearly require calling upon the expertise of a professional—fixing a car or fixing a broken leg for example. So, what does a psychotherapist fix? If you can't answer that question, then maybe you should at least think about it before committing yourself (and your money) to consulting a professional.

Let's imagine a Non Governmental Organisation sends 5,000 volunteer water-supply engineers to a developing country where most people have no access to running water within a two hours walk of their homes. What would we expect to see a year later? Surely, more people having access to clean running water in or near their home.

What would we deduce if a year later even fewer people had access to drinking water?

This is somewhat the case with psychologists and sociologists. Increasing the number of experts has not led to a reduction in the number of problems. Maybe it's just a case of not knowing how screwed up we really are until we have the required experts to tell us.

When someone feels they "need" counselling or has been told, "You really need to see someone," they commonly have an issue that causes great emotional suffering. The person doesn't want to suffer any more but feels incapable of fixing the problem herself. She feels she needs help from an expert.

However, if you ask a person why they are in therapy, most of the time they will give you the wrong answer. "Because I'm depressed all the time." Wrong answer—you can be as depressed as you want without seeing a therapist. "Because I suffer from terrible migraine headaches, and the pills don't work any more." Wrong answer—you can suffer the torture of a migraine headache without seeing a therapist.

Usually, the person will show some irritation at this point, and say, "You know what I mean. I want somebody to stop all the suffering." That's an improvement, but we're still not there.

~

After a few years of my hypnotherapy practice, I began cutting to the chase with a new client at the beginning of their first session by asking just one question. It was always the same: "If you didn't have problem 'X' what would you be able to do that you can't do now?"

I know my client is sitting in front of me because they want to experience life differently. Rarely, however, have they put thought into what that difference would be in practical terms. (I should point out here that sometimes my insistence on obtaining an answer to this question meant I never saw the person again. Try studying Psychology 101 if you want to know why.)

Mrs Cavin was about forty years old. She looked pale and tired and had difficulty finding her words when she sat down in front of me. She told me she suffered from agoraphobia. For the previous year, she had been so terrified of leaving her house a neighbour had to take her children to and from school and she had to do all of her shopping online. In order to attend her appointment with me, she admitted she had needed a large brandy. Or two.

I start with my question. "What, precisely, would you be able to do that you can't do today if you didn't suffer from agoraphobia?"

She looked at me uncomprehendingly, wondering if it's a trick question.

(Of course it is I want to tell her, but I resist.)

"I'd be able to go out. Wouldn't I?"

"Yes, of course. But why do you want to be able to go out?"

After a pause, she decides to play the game. "It's horrid being a prisoner in your own home. I sometimes feel like I'm going crazy.

And I know I am driving my family crazy."

"OK. So now we know what you don't want. But we still don't know what you do want. Tell me what's so great about going out? Where would you go?"

By now she's probably thinking there is something seriously wrong with me, but she answers anyway. "There is one thing I am dreading. Summer will be here in a few weeks. I used to love going to the beach. Just lying there, soaking up the sun, splashing around in the sea.... You know the kind of thing. What makes it worse is that we only live half a mile from the beach, but I know I can't go there."

I alter the course of my questioning.

"So, you're saying that you'd like to feel happy about going to the beach?"

A tearful nod of the head, "Yes, but—"

I cut her off with the next question, nudging a box of Kleenex tissues towards her: "When was the last time you felt happy?"

I wait for the sobs to subside. She continues, "I almost can't remember. It was probably during a day on the beach over two years ago."

Now comes the killer question that will change everything.

"Can you remember what it felt like, being happy on the beach?"

After a moment, she puts on the expected dreamy look, the muscular tensions melting away from her face. Her mouth curls up in a half-smile. She is looking up and away somewhere, not at me. This is also expected.

I let her enjoy the moment for about a minute, then I spoil everything by asking, "Do you have any idea how you might be able to feel that happiness again?"

The smile disappears.

She looks at me a little resentfully. "I sometimes think that I'll never be happy again. It's as if I've forgotten how to do feeling happy."

Then I do something cruel. I say nothing. I let the silence drag on. I am good at this. Silences don't bother me. Maybe I have missed my vocation as a Freudian psychoanalyst or a Trappist monk.

When she can bear it no longer, she says, "What?"

I ask her to repeat the last sentence she said.

"I don't know how to be happy any more. Was that it?"

It wasn't, but it's close enough to make no difference.

My next question alone is worth what she's paid all the other counsellors: "So, what were you feeling when you were remembering your last day on the beach?"

"Er, warm and happy?"

"But you don't do 'warm and happy' any more."

Gotcha!

And I haven't even started talking about hypnosis.

By this point in the story you may have recognised elements of Neuro-Linguistic Programming, Cognitive Behavioural Therapy, and Transactional Analysis. You may have also spotted elements of pattern interrupt, surprise, and contradiction which we spoke about in an earlier chapter. And you would be right. So, what?

Maybe you're thinking I played a trick on her. Just like I lied to my pupil, Jamel. You would be right there too.

It wasn't the first time Mrs Cavin had been able to express herself and talk freely about her problem. She was no longer just talking it through. I correctly guessed she had already used all the synonyms for "suffering" a thousand times to many different therapists.

Too much getting things off your chest can be bad for your soul.

Instead, I got her to talk to me about what she would be able to do in the future and linked it to what she had already done in the past. For one minute she experienced "warmth and happiness." Right there in my office. In the *hic et nunc.* As far as she was concerned, I hadn't even started doing my hypnotherapy.

I made her pay anyway.

Just another shock and we'll be through with Mrs Cavin.

At that point, I said, "That will be all for today. If you feel you'd like to come back, you can call to make an appointment."

That was it.

So, what was actually going on there? Are these the slick tricks of modern psychotherapy? Yes. And no. After all, she could have purchased a self-help book and read about this kind of approach.

To understand what was really happening, we have to return to the magic of a therapeutic relationship. She came to me asking for help. My ad in the Yellow Pages had told her I was offering help.

The fact I helped her in an unexpected way is of no importance if you discount the benefits of a healthy shock.

I, Richard Morgan, bearer of the title Hypnotherapist, enabled Mrs Cavin to realise the impossible: feel happy.

OK, so it was only for one minute, but it doesn't matter. Mrs Cavin was convinced that nothing could make her happy. I showed her she was wrong. And that changed everything.

I would not have helped her by explaining how I was going to proceed to make her feel happy again. There are many insecure or incompetent therapists who make the mistake of giving lengthy explanations. When they do this, they are just reassuring themselves or trying to make the session last for the promised number of minutes. Alas, they often justify themselves by saying it is in the patient's interest to understand what is going on.

But why? There is no good answer.

~

OK, OK, I hear you. You want to know if Mrs Cavin called to make a further appointment with me.

No, she didn't. But guess who I saw on the beach a few weeks later?

Oh, and before I forget—do you need therapy?

Frankly, I have no idea.

CHAPTER 7

Evolution and Happy Lapses

According to the *New England Journal of Medicine*, twenty-seven percent of men develop an inguinal hernia at some point during their lifetime. [12] Usually this occurs before their first birthday or after the age of fifty. Inguinal hernias are caused when tissue protrudes through a weakness or an opening in the muscles of the abdominal wall.

If you're curious, like me, you might like to know what kind of "tissue" is protruding, and why there is a weakness or an opening in the muscles of the abdominal wall in the first place.

With a little more research I discovered the testes of a human male form within the abdomen. Later during gestation, the testes move down to the scrotum and have to pass through the abdominal wall to do so. This passage leaves two weak spots in the wall. These spots can herniate, allowing the intestines to slither out under the skin. Herniation both strangles the intestine and cuts off/slows the blood flow to the affected testis. Without surgery, this can lead to excruciating pain and death.

That answers that question.

Evolution is defined as:

> Random Mutations + Natural Selection = the Appearance of New Species [13]

Genetic mutations occur for mostly unknown reasons, which is why we call them "random." However, there is nothing random about natural selection. If a mutation confers a survival advantage in the current environment, it is kept in the gene pool and it becomes part of the organism. If a mutation lowers the chances of survival, it will be selected against. This is because the individuals will fail to survive.

Natural selection hangs on to whatever works.

Take, for example, the collared doves that come to feed on my balcony. They are scared of anything moving that's bigger than a doughnut, including me. And I'm only there to serve them breakfast.

Are they paranoid or are they just normal collared doves doing what a normal collared dove does?

Imagine the behaviours of two different sets of collared doves: one set has the instinct to flee anything that moves, and the other treats everything that moves as a potential source of breakfast. Which set is more likely to survive? The cowards, of course. The others would have very rapidly become somebody else's breakfast.

For a species to survive, a sufficient number of individuals need to reach a reproductive age and then do some actual reproducing before shuffling off this mortal coil. Failure to survive spells the extinction of the species. So does failing to reproduce.

Due to the relatively late age when hernias occur, there has been plenty of time for the male to reproduce. Evolution has done its job. Those two weak spots in the male abdominal wall do not affect the survival of humankind and so still remain. Which is bad news for men, for we would rather have the odds of suffering an inguinal hernia a little lower.

Life (survival) and the quality of life are two distinct, unrelated issues. Live. Mature. Reproduce. And that's it from an evolutionary perspective. As long as babies keep on being born and living on into adulthood to make more babies, homo sapiens continues to roll along.

Comfort is not a selection criterion.

Dang!

~

Have you ever tried reasoning with a baby? If you have children, of course you have. Typically, you attempt doing so in a sleep-deprived haze at 3am when you still have an outside chance of another four hours sleep, baby willing. The thing is, no amount of clever reasoning will work, for it is impossible to reason with a baby. They will continue to express any feeling of discomfort without any consideration of the time or your lack of sleep. This is because we are born without the ability to analyse. A baby's brain doesn't process the information it is receiving, it simply accepts it uncritically.

At what stage does the growing child become capable of saying, "Whoa. Hang on. What's going on here?" There are various theories concerning the "age of reason" but most people eventually get there.

There are many benefits to a baby's lack of critical thinking. When you require a mother figure for food, cleaning, warmth, hugs, and even burping, unquestioning trust is very helpful. When there is so much to learn about the world, from how to walk to how to speak, being able to absorb new information swiftly and without analysis is extremely useful.

However, like many survival features, there is a downside to a child's uncritical trust and learning. Some would call it gullibility. Others blind faith. Suggestibility is another name. It is an interesting state of mind because it can be created, albeit temporarily, within adults. Hypnotherapists and used car salesman know how to do this. In fact, this state of suggestibility is present in all therapies. Why?

Because a therapeutic relationship is fundamentally regressive.

A plea for help meets an offer of help. A weakness meets a strength. The horizontal meets the vertical.

That's precisely how you started life.

When somebody who is suffering makes a plea for help, they are saying, "I can't do this by myself." Just as we all communicate at the beginning of our lives, "I can't feed myself, I can't keep myself warm, I can't change myself." This child-like dependency is not like milk teeth, which once lost are gone forever to be replaced by costly dental treatment. When evolution selected the powers of critical thinking, they were *added* to developing mental processes.

They did not delete the potential for becoming helpless again.

Saying, "Please help me" re-activates our early mental state. Temporarily, we suspend all critical thinking and regress to how we used to relate to our mother. This includes the ability to receive and assimilate new information without question.

Most people are reluctant to admit they can lapse into regressive modes of behaviour, not realising that lovers do it all the time quite unashamedly. In English, they call each other "baby" and worse. In French, a term of endearment is *"mon choux"*—my cabbage. (Don't ask me why.)

Whatever the therapist's or healer's language or method, his presence is saying, "Mummy's here. Everything's going to be alright. I'll take care of you."

Remember, Serge's terse formula, "I'll take care of it"?

The marabou who claims to solve all problems is adopting a position of maternal omnipotence.

The hypnotherapist is quite flagrantly "lulling" his patient. He probably doesn't call his patient "baby," but the tone of his voice and the language he chooses to use, all say the same thing.

Practitioners of manual therapy do not tend to use words. However, they interact with our body to communicate the same motherly care. "I'm here. I'm holding you."

Why do we still have this regressive potential? Quite simply because it does not interfere with survival or reproduction. It is evolutionarily neutral.

~

The human brain has developed what is often called "higher" faculties. These create a sensation of self-consciousness which allows an individual to take stock of his situation over and above the immediate survival and reproductive imperatives. We can think about things that are not present or perceptible. Above all, we can think about the future, and what it may hold.

What does that give us?

Books, music, and poetry.

Scientific and technological advancement.

Religion and philosophy.

A sense of humour.

Brotherly love.

Self-sacrifice.

Condoms and birth control pills.

And a whole truck-load of other non-essential stuff from a "survive and reproduce" viewpoint. Evolutionary scientists have various explanations and names for this:

"Evolutionary misfiring."

"Spandrels."

"Exaptation."

"By-products."

And more recently "neo-purposes" or "neo-goals" as an accidental extension of "archi-purposes."

I prefer the substantially less scientific term, "happy accidents."

The one that interests us here is the happy accident to regress. To be able to reach out and say "help."

Sometimes this calling out for succour is institutionalised. Take a look at people in some Christian churches "praising the Lord." Arms stretched up in the air. Reaching out to be picked up. Same gestures. Same messages.

I'm small, you're big; pick me up and take care of me.

~

The truly amazing thing is that the capacity to help (like a parent) or to ask for help (like a baby) is universal. Helping somebody through a difficult period does not require diplomas, white coats, or a lack of scruples. Asking for help does not entail losing one's dignity. You always suspected that to be true.

But...

Because there's always a "but," isn't there?

CHAPTER 8

Placebo/Nocebo. A Science of Care?

To take my blood pressure, my doctor used an old-fashioned sphygmomanometer. First, she would fasten a vicious cuff around my upper arm. Then she would tighten the cuff by pumping an air bulb, stopping just before my arm dropped off my body. When she was satisfied that I was already having visions of needing to learn to play Ravel's piano concerto for left hand, she would stop pumping. She would hook her stethoscope into her ears, and turn and open the air-valve, slowly releasing the air, while positioning the chestpiece of the stethoscope in the crook of my paralysed arm. (Yes, it's really called the chestpiece. I didn't make that up.) As you may be able to tell, I love being attended to by doctors and nurses.

My doctor doesn't wear a white coat. And in any case, I wouldn't have called it "White Coat Syndrome" when she took my blood pressure. My doctor was a young and very attractive woman. I am a relatively normal male. So, I decided to call my high blood pressure result the "Mammary Proximity Syndrome." This kicked in when she would block my forearm between her upper arm and her, er... chest. How could that not affect my blood pressure? I would ask myself that question every time, but I never said anything in case she stopped doing it.

Men! Really!

She listened and watched the mercury level dropping while I tried to think about Queen and country.

"It's still too high," she said, "165 and 120. We're going to have to try a combination medicine."

The word "combination" made me feel a little nervous, but Doctor knows best.

Years ago, this particular doctor had given me strict instructions to avoid reading the patient information leaflet with any medicines she prescribed for me. This is because she knew I was highly suggestible. I only had to read the terrifying list of possible side effects, and within a few hours I would start experiencing things like nausea, dizziness, a dry mouth, and the odd hallucination. I never seemed to suffer any side effects when I didn't read the insert. Some of the medicines even seemed to help me.

Yes, I know, I shouldn't have read the leaflet this time either. I resisted the temptation for as long as I could, but in the end, I opened the box of pills, removed the insert and started reading. I skipped all the harmless stuff, including the warning for pregnant women, and concentrated on the possible side effects.

Reading the long, terrifying list made Stephen King novels seem like bed-time fairy tales in comparison.

Are you ready?

Here we go. (The print on patient information leaflets is always painfully small, so in the interests of authenticity I have reduced the font size.)

Severe allergic reactions. The signs may include sudden onset of:
Swelling of your face, lips, tongue, or throat. This may make it difficult to swallow.
Severe or sudden swelling of your hands, feet, or ankles.
Difficulty breathing.
Severe itching of the skin (with raised lumps).

Severe liver problems. The signs may include:
Yellowing of your skin or eyes, dark coloured urine or a loss of appetite.

Other possible side effects:
Common (may affect up to 1 in 10 people)
Headache.
Feeling dizzy or light-headed, especially if you stand up quickly.
Fainting.
Diarrhoea.
Being sick (vomiting).
Cough.
Kidney problems (shown in a blood test).

Uncommon (may affect up to 1 in 100 people)
Mood changes including feeling depressed.
Tingling feeling such as 'pins and needles'.
Spinning feeling (vertigo).
Changes in the way things taste.
Difficulty in sleeping.
Heart attack or stroke.
Unusual heartbeat.
Change of colour in your fingers or toes.
Runny nose.
Feeling sick (nausea).
Stomach pain and indigestion.

Changes in blood tests that check how the liver is working.
Rash.
Itching.
Being unable to get an erection (impotence).
Feeling weak.
Feeling tired.
Increased levels of certain substances in your blood (urea, creatinine, or potassium).

Rare (may affect up to 1 in 1,000 people)
Changes to some of the cells or other parts of your blood. The signs may include feeling tired and pale skin.
Feeling confused.
Changes in the way things smell.
Dry mouth.
Skin rash with dark red, raised, itchy bumps (hives).
Hair loss (alopecia).
Psoriasis (a skin problem).
Infection of the blood.
Kidney failure.
Enlarged breasts in men.
Syndrome of inappropriate antidiuretic hormone secretion (SIADH).
Low levels of sodium in the blood, which may cause weakness, tiredness, headache, feeling sick, being sick (vomiting) and cramps.

Very rare (may affect up to 1 in 10,000 people)
Problems with your bone marrow or a reduced number of blood cells and/or platelets in your blood. You may notice tiredness, an infection (which may be serious), fever, feeling breathless or that you bruise or bleed more easily.
Swollen glands (lymph nodes).
Increased immune response (autoimmune disease).
Low levels of sugar in your blood (hypoglycaemia). The signs may include feeling hungry or weak, sweating and a fast heartbeat.
Suddenly feeling wheezy or short of breath (bronchospasm).
Lung inflammation (which may make you feel breathless).
Sinusitis (a feeling of pain and fullness behind your cheeks and eyes).
Eosinophilic pneumonia. The signs include a combination of the

following: sinusitis, feeling like you have flu, feeling more and more breathless, pain in the area of your stomach or gut, skin rash, a feeling of 'pins and needles' or numbness of your arms or legs.
Inflammation of the pancreas. This causes moderate to severe pain in the stomach.
Swelling of the lining of the gut. This may cause sudden stomach pain, diarrhoea, or make you be sick (vomit).
Sweating.
Severe skin disorder or rash. The symptoms include redness, blistering and peeling of the skin which may develop quickly and may include blistering in the mouth and nose.
Passing less water (urine) than normal or passing no water.

Not known (frequency cannot be estimated from the available data)
Seeing, feeling or hearing things that are not there (hallucinations).
Flushing of your skin.
Possible side effects with hydrochlorothiazide (frequency not known).
Inflammation of a salivary gland.
A reduced number of blood cells and/or platelets in your blood. You may notice tiredness, an infection (which may be serious), fever, feeling breathless or that you bruise or bleed more easily.
Loss of appetite.
An increase in the amount of sugar (glucose) in your blood (hyperglycaemia).
Sugar in your urine.
An increase in the amount of uric acid in your blood.
Altered levels of substances in your blood (for example low sodium and potassium). You may notice muscle weakness, thirst, 'pins and needles', cramps or feeling sick.
Raised or high levels of fats in your blood (including cholesterol).
Feeling restless.
Depression.
Difficulty sleeping.
Tingling feelings such as 'pins and needles'.
Feeling light-headed.
Changes to your vision that can make things look yellow.
Problems with your sight for a short time.

Severe eye pain with redness and sudden blurred vision. If you have a suddenly painful red eye tell your doctor immediately; you may need treatment to avoid permanent loss of vision.
A spinning feeling (vertigo).
Feeling faint (especially when standing up).
Damage to blood vessels causing red or purple spots in the skin.
Difficulty breathing. You may feel breathless if your lungs get inflamed or have fluid on them.
Stomach irritation.
Diarrhoea.
Constipation.
Inflammation of the pancreas. This causes moderate to severe pain in the stomach.
Yellowing of your skin or the whites of your eyes (jaundice).
Skin problems including rash caused by sensitivity to sunlight, rash, severe rash that develops quickly with blistering or peeling of the skin and possibly blistering in the mouth, activating or worsening of existing lupus conditions or appearance of unusual skin reactions.
Muscle cramps and muscle weakness.
Kidney problems which may be severe (shown in blood tests).
Fever.
Weakness.

After reading all that I was left with the impression that high blood pressure seemed a safer option. Depression and seeing everything yellow? The risks of strokes, heart attacks, and kidney failure seemed laughable in comparison. I decided I would take the pills all the same and resolved to start the treatment the very next day.

When I woke up the next morning, I went into the kitchen to prepare myself a cup of tea.

As I was waiting for the kettle to boil, I carefully placed my new pill on the kitchen table next to my cup and teaspoon to make sure I didn't forget to take it.

I put the tea-bag in the cup, drowned it in boiling water, then went to check my email while it was brewing.

Barely half an hour after drinking my tea and taking the pill, I started feeling a little dizzy. That was definitely on the list somewhere. A few minutes later I felt waves of nausea sweeping over me, and I definitely felt my heartbeat accelerate. But what really made me panic was when I started seeing things yellow! Well, yellowish.

I was feeling really unwell. I was worried. I thought a glass of cold water might make me feel better, so I staggered to the kitchen with great difficulty. I had to hold on to things to avoid losing my balance and falling over.

Since I know just how suggestible I am, I said to myself, "Calm down Richard, it's all in your imagination." But it didn't help. I made it to the kitchen and the first thing I saw was the table where I had left my tea to brew.

The teaspoon was still there.

And so was the pill.

I hadn't even taken it. But I still got the undesirable side effects.

~

Everybody has heard about the placebo effect. Welcome to the nocebo effect. It's what happens when harmless or inert substances make you feel ill. (Even if you don't take them!) Much less fun than the placebo effect where a pill containing nothing at all can make you feel better.

How do the placebo/nocebo effects actually work? What are the neurobiological mechanisms which enable a thought or a belief to bring about physiological changes? Does anybody know?

Thinking about all the fun I have with spine-chilling patient information leaflets, I realised it was time to do some research.

I discovered a fascinating article written by Cara Feinberg in a 2013 edition of Harvard Magazine. It was entitled, *The Placebo Phenomenon: An ingenious researcher finds the real ingredients of "fake" medicine.* [14] In the article, she discusses the work and findings of Ted Kaptchuk, a researcher of placebo effects at the Program in Placebo Studies and the Therapeutic Encounter headquartered at Beth Israel Deaconess Medical Center in Boston. This research program had been originally created by Kaptchuk and his colleagues from several Harvard-affiliated hospitals.

Cara Feinberg writes:

> For the last 15 years, Kaptchuk and his fellow researchers have been dissecting placebo interventions—treatments that, prior to the 1990s, had been studied largely as foils to "real" drugs. To prove a medicine is effective, pharmaceutical companies must show not only that their drug has the desired effects, but that the effects are significantly greater than those of a placebo control group. Both groups often show healing results, Kaptchuk explains, yet for years, "We were struggling to increase drug effects while no one was trying to increase the placebo effect."

This looked promising. In order to increase an effect, you need to know how it works. I read on.

> Explanations for the phenomenon come from fields across the scientific map—clinical science, psychology, anthropology, biology, social economics, neuroscience. Disregarding the knowledge that placebo treatments can affect certain ailments, Kaptchuk says, "is like ignoring a huge chunk of healthcare." As caregivers, "we should be using every tool in the box."

Yes!

Later in the article, Feinberg quotes from email correspondence she'd had with Fabrizio Benedetti, a professor of physiology and neuroscience at the University of Turin Medical School in Italy. He also is a member of the six-strong group on Placebo of the Mind-Brain-Behavior Initiative at Harvard University, and a consultant for the Placebo Project at the U.S. National Institute of Health.

> "What we 'placebo neuroscientists'... have learned [is] that therapeutic rituals move a lot of molecules in the patients' brain, and these molecules are the very same as those activated by the drugs we give in routine clinical practice," Benedetti wrote in an email. "In other words, rituals and drugs use the very same biochemical pathways to influence the patient's brain." It's those advances in "hard science," he added, that have given placebo research a legitimacy it never enjoyed before.

Imaging technology such as Positron Emission Tomography (PET) scans and Functional Magnetic Resonance Imaging (FMRI) "show biological evidence that minds actually change" writes Feinberg. (For the purposes of this topic, I did not object to the mind/brain conflation.) What change do these images actually reveal? And what does this activity achieve?

I discovered, "the placebo-activated endogenous opioid systems have been shown to have a somatotopic organisation." [15]

That mouthful of a sentence may have caused momentary mind blank, so let me break it down. "Endogenous" refers to something created from within. An "endogenous opioid system" is a system in the brain which secretes chemicals called opioids. These produce morphine-like effects as well as having a similar effect to the opiates you can buy from your local, street-corner dealer. As for "somatotopic," any word that contains "somat" refers to the physical body. A well-known example is psychosomatic, where the mind (psycho) actually affects the body (somatic). "Somatotopic organisation" is fancy-scientific-speak for saying there are measurable changes in what is going on in the (physical) brain caused by a placebo.

Therefore, a placebo activates the production of an opioid, a chemical which inhibits certain brain activities. Could one of the activities include the use of the critical faculties?

To a certain extent Kaptchuk and his colleagues are discovering how brain activities are modified. However, the last paragraph in Feinberg's article is very telling:

> In order to legitimise his findings to mainstream practitioners, the results must be expertly quantified, [Kaptchuk] acknowledges. "We have to transform the art of medicine into the science of care."

To my cynical mind, that sounded a lot like, "Doctors will be more interested in caring if it's scientific." But that is a different issue. Maybe a different book.

I wonder whether it will be possible for Kaptchuk and his

colleagues to detect similarities between an undeveloped infant brain and an adult brain experiencing a moment of regression? The results from that research could give them the basis for a "science of care," and doctors would feel legitimised in really caring for their patients.

Or they could just read this book.

CHAPTER 9

What Actually Happens in Psychotherapy (But Your Therapist Never Tells You)?

"You can cure phobias, can't you?" she asked anxiously.

I avoided answering her question directly. "Yes, people have come to see me with phobia problems and after a few sessions told me their phobia had disappeared."

Doesn't that prove I can cure phobias?

Well, no.

Firstly, before making any wild claims about any kind of "cure," I would need to see the person at least five years later. This would confirm whether some sort of lasting cure had taken place.

Secondly, I don't even know what it would mean to say I had cured anybody of anything. If my friend wants to drive from Toulouse to

Paris but discovers his car battery is flat, he might ask me if I had a set of jump leads. If I then link his ailing battery to the healthy one in my car, start my engine, and keep it running until his engine starts, he will at least be able to drive to the end of the road. He might even manage to drive the 600km to Paris. However, does that mean I am in a position to claim he got to Paris on account of me? If I made that sort of claim, and my friend got killed in an accident on the motorway, I suppose I would have to say it was my fault. No, I could only pride myself on having recharged his battery. His successful arrival in Paris was all down to many other factors outside of my control or input.

Correlation is not causation. But I was not about to explain all that to 38-year-old Chantal. Not that I wanted to hide anything but simply because it would be unhelpful to her at that point.

Chantal was a primary school teacher. Her parents were farmers. Salt of the earth kind of people. She had been the first person ever from her family to go to college and obtain a degree.

She explained to me she was terrified of thunder and lightning. She said she could not remember a time in her life when she did not have this fear. However, this fear had worsened over the past couple of years. It had got to the point where if the sky looked a bit overcast, she had to keep glancing out of the window to see if a storm was brewing. She would do this even in front of her class of 8-year-olds. This issue had become such a handicap, she was thinking about resigning from teaching.

Her fear had engendered a fear of fear.

She had read somewhere that by using hypnosis it was possible to unearth early memories of events that were at the origin of phobias. I did not confirm this, but neither did I contradict what she said. I simply complied with her desire to experience age regression.

After two sessions she announced her phobia had disappeared.

Her explanation—the one that she would retain and share with people who enquired about her visits to the "hypnotist"—was that she relived several experiences from when she had been five or six-years-old while in a hypnotic "trance." Whenever there was a thunderstorm, her mother would hide in a cubbyhole under the stairs, dragging her daughter with her. The traumatising aspect of this for Chantal was seeing her mother in a state of panic. "Maman," who should have been strong for her daughter, trembled and blubbered like a terrified child with every rumble of thunder or flash of lightning.

Chantal had always known her mother suffered from this phobia. She assumed her own phobia had been picked up through her mother's influence. It sounded logical, didn't it? After reliving these experiences, Chantal realised that while her mother had been scared of thunder and lightning, Chantal herself was frightened of *behaving like her mother*—especially in front of her pupils.

It then became a classic case of a fear being dissipated by having been identified and confronted. She was able to say to herself things like, "Hey! I'm not my mother. Why should I be frightened of having the same reactions as her? I am not an uneducated, superstitious country girl."

This all sounds like fairly basic therapy stuff. Nothing startling. No revelations there. Chantal was able to enter safely into a regressive relationship with me and then recognise and deal with a problem.

The one thing I did not tell Chantal was we had no proof she had recuperated *genuine* memories. They could have been invented or at least reshaped over the years. All our memories, even those from yesterday, are liable to be imperfect. We are much more likely to retain the emotions of an event rather than specific details. And even that is only a supposition. Maybe Chantal had never been in a cubby hole with her mother although it seems likely she could have been.

~

Previous life therapy claims that some problems we experience in this life could be due to traumas experienced in a previous life. In order to access the origins and possible cause of the problems the patient needs to relive the past life. That's the theory.

One patient, a woman in her early fifties, believed this would solve the problem of her recurring migraine headaches. Like most of the people who consulted me, she had first consulted her GP and a handful of specialists with no results. The hypnotherapist was typically a last resort.

When talking about her migraine headaches, she said the most unpleasant feature was a sharp and persistent stabbing pain just above her left eye. I duly noted this on a pad of paper. For some people, seeing the therapist note their words gives them the impression they are being listened to and taken seriously. Others need to have your full attention through eye-to-eye contact. Some therapists make notes just to avoid such eye-to-eye contact.

I used a fairly standard "previous life regression" technique. My patient soon started speaking in a masculine voice. We were able to determine that he/she was a farm worker. He/she spoke with an east country accent. We were later able to situate this in the mid-18th century though the exact geographical location remained a mystery.

She/he told me that he had no time to stop and talk—there was work to be done. He and another labourer were stacking hay in a barn, using large pitch-forks.

All of a sudden, my patient let out a piercing scream, doubled up and clasped her hands over—yes, you've guessed it—her left eye. The co-worker had accidentally stabbed him/her in the eye with his pitchfork. (Later my patient described feeling warm blood trickling between her fingers!)

Shuttling back and forth between different periods in this "previous life" we learned that the eye was lost, but the farm labourer survived. There was a lot of weeping and other emotional phenomena that are sometimes called abreactions. On returning to the "present time" my patient said she felt a huge sensation of relief.

One month later, she returned to see me. She told me she had not experienced any attacks of migraines since her previous visit. But there was more. She expressed a sense of liberation in her life in general. She certainly appeared much more laid back and relaxed than when she had first come to see me. Of course, there could be several explanations for that.

I didn't see her again, but for over a year I got a lot of positive feedback through all the people she had recommended to come and see me. They were all migraine sufferers.

~

Now, it just so happens I don't "believe" in reincarnation. But I am convinced of the amazingly creative powers of the imagination. It would seem that certain circumstances can be brought about to unleash these creative powers to help resolve a person's issues.

We had no actual proof Chantal had been holed up with her mother during storms even though it was possible. In the case of the victim of a careless pitchforker, there could never be any evidence at all of a "previous life." But does this matter?

It could be argued that two people who had suffered a great deal in their lives, appeared to have been relieved of their suffering.

Again, we have to ask: what is going on here?

As Dr Nick Read points out:

> The effects of new psychiatric treatments are not easy to assess. There are no measurable end points like inflammation, blood pressure, blood sugar levels. There's just patient testimony. 'Yes, I'm feeling much better, thank you.' Good results may be more due to the care and attention of the doctors and nurses than any effect of the treatment. It all depends how you ask the question and what statistical methods are applied. Powerful advocates and suggestible patients can still produce 'effective' treatments. Perhaps that's the nature of the mind; it's confidence and faith that heals the traumatised psyche—and there are many routes to that. [16]

In this book, I dare to go beyond "it's confidence and faith that heals the traumatised psyche." Even the most sceptical of my patients had to at least exercise enough confidence and faith to come into my office and expose their problems to me. Maybe, this is enough. I can't say one hundred percent one way or the other. What I do know, and to which I alluded to earlier, is that the hypnotist was often towards the end of the chain of specialists a patient had visited. Why hadn't their confidence and faith healed them long before coming to see me?

For perhaps half of my patients, I wasn't the end of the line either, just another attempt at healing along the way.

What your psychotherapist will not tell you, often because he is unaware of the fact himself, is that all forms of therapy, without exception, rely heavily on establishing the same regressive relationship.

There are no exceptions.

This does not mean that all therapies or healing methods will produce positive results. Not everyone gets better, anywhere. Not in the traditional doctor's surgery, or on the hypnotist's couch, or under the onslaught of a marabou's incantations.

In the two cases I have cited in this chapter, we again find what I see as the two basic, essential ingredients for healing broken lives: a demand for help encountering an offer of help. The relationship which is formed through this interaction can reproduce in the person asking for help the receptive, uncritical helplessness of a baby.

Why could this be important for you? How could it potentially be life-changing? This is what you will discover in the remaining chapters.

CHAPTER 10

Positively Bullshit

One cold Monday evening I was attending a Choro workshop in Toulouse with my recently acquired bandolim—a Brazilian mandolin. This was a structured class where anyone could turn up with an instrument and participate in learning the "language" of Choro. Regardless of the number of musicians, we all sit in a circle to make eye contact easy. This is important, for after one person starts us off, everyone takes turns joining in the improvised melody.

Choro is a popular style of instrumental music that originated in Brazil during the late 19th century. The name "Choro" actually means "cry" or "lament," which is ironic, for the music itself is a lively, varied mix of styles that is wonderful to behold. It is often played in relaxed, informal get-togethers known as a "roda de Choro." Roda literally means a "circle of people."

On this particular evening there were guitars, pandeiros, accordions, trumpets, clarinets, saxophones, one cavaquinho, my bandolim, and three flutes. That is, until the pause. When we all took our places again after a short break, I noticed there were only two flutes now being played. Looking around, I spotted Didier, our missing flautist, sitting alone in a corner. He looked down and stayed there until the end of the evening.

Before packing away my music and my bandolim, I went over to him and said, "You're not looking too good, Didier."

"Yeah, problems at work, problems at home—"

Abruptly, he stood up and went outside.

When I left a few minutes later, I saw Didier outside. He was leaning against a wall, rolling a cigarette. He looked up at me, his expression conveying a tacit desire to talk. He had obviously been waiting for me.

"Thanks, for noticing, Richard. I'm sorry I walked away like that, but things are pretty rough at the moment. I didn't want to break down in front of everybody."

I just touched his arm and said, "Well, I'm here again now if..." I deliberately didn't finish the sentence, leaving him the space to pick up the conversation again... or not.

Then it all came out. The word he used the most frequently was "tensions." Tensions at home, tensions at work.

I listened. I didn't put on a therapist's benign, understanding half smile. (Whenever I see that, it makes me want to break teeth.) I was just present.

After a couple of minutes, he tried to pull himself together, perhaps embarrassed at having said too much. "I was in therapy last year, and the therapist taught me how to look on the positive side of things, so that's what I'm trying to do. It helps."

"I beg your pardon. 'The positive side of things'?"

"Yeah, there's always something positive to take hold of—"

"Bullshit."

He looked at me, eyebrows raised in surprise.

"Did you say...?"

"Yes. Bullshit."

"What do you mean?"

Picking up on his therapist's words, I said, "Have you ever tried to tell a man who's drowning that he ought to look on the positive side of things?"

"Yeah, no, but I'm not drowning...."

A few moment's pause.

I remained silent. Helping a person in great pain or distress to identify positive aspects of his life to hang on to can sometimes be the very best thing to do. However, it is not something that always works in all circumstances.

Didier took a drag on his hand-rolled cigarette, then raised his eyes to watch the smoke coalesce in the icy air and languidly drift away.

"You're right. It is bullshit. I'd always had the feeling that it was a bit dumb. And, yes, I do feel like I am drowning. When I can't find anything positive to grasp on to, I just feel guilty that I'm not making enough of an effort. Yep. Bullshit." he said, nodding his head in typical Gallic fashion, as if agreeing with himself. Then I saw there was a smile slowly creasing his cheeks. He started chuckling. "It really is bullshit, isn't it? Fuck—it feels so good to have someone agree with me. Thank you for that, Richard."

We never spoke of his "problems" again. The following Monday, he played his flute all evening. He was smiling most of the time. Just at one point, he looked across the table at me and said quietly, "Fucking bullshit, right?"

~

As a general rule, we don't like revealing our personal problems to others. Equally, many people are uneasy about listening to somebody talk about their difficulties. And when it comes to expressing our feelings as well as our issues, well, we usually behave like the collared doves on my balcony. We assume a threat, a danger.

In fact, collared doves are smarter than people in one way. They can allow their hunger to stifle their instinctive flight reaction in certain circumstances. The collared doves I told you about earlier eventually ended up eating out of my hand. Before long they were visibly fatter than their pals.

Why are we so reluctant to share our problems?

Because it's just "not done" in polite society? Why?

Because we're frightened of what the other person may think of us? Why?

Because we're sure the other person would not understand?

How can we be sure?

Because the context isn't right? What difference does a framed diploma on a wall make?

Because some things are just too painful to put into words?

Probably all of those and more.

Françoise Dolto, the French psychoanalyst, said, *"Mettre des mots sur ce qu'on éprouve, aussi bien dans la tendresse que dans la haine, c'est cela qui est humain."* "Using words to express feelings, either in affection or in hatred, is just being human." [17]

We need words. And we need silences.

Astonishing things can happen when we express our need for help. People often start to feel better after making an appointment with a counsellor, even before setting foot in his office. Why? Because they have dared to say, "Please help me."

You may be thinking, "That's all well and good. It is a positive step to decide to seek out a professional counsellor, or a foot masseur, or a hypnotist. But you can't confide your worries to just anyone on the street."

Why not?

Let's look at why most people prefer to avoid hearing about other people's existential woes. It all comes down to how listening to a person's pain will draw our attention to our own pain before we can empathise.

"How are you today?"

"Well, I didn't sleep too well and I've got a bit of a headache."

"I understand. I really do. I had a headache once that lasted for three years. The most terrible pain you can imagine. I tried everything, but nothing helped. It ruined my life. The excruciating pounding in my head almost drove me crazy. I even tried a brain transplant, but the new brain hurt even more than the old one. I paid a fortune to see the Queen's personal osteopath... blah, blah, blah."

Giving an honest answer to how we're feeling tends to turn the conversation into being about someone else's problem. So, what we generally hear, in every country in the world is:

"How are you today?"

"Fine thanks. How are you?"

"Yes, I'm good."

Everybody is comfortable with that. To a certain extent.

Freud said that everybody should be psychoanalysed. (I suppose that getting people to believe that was good for business. You?) What I am saying is that we all have the potential to be an occasional therapist, counsellor, or magician.

White coats, diplomas, or skilful advertising copy written by or for the unscrupulous are no guarantee of effective help. All of us actually have the potential to make a difference in a person's life.

It's just nobody ever told you this before.

- Fact: We all need some kind of help or support at some point in our lives.
- Fact: Fear cuts us off from each other, sometimes even seriously isolating us.

- Fact: Many things we aspire to are on "the other side of fear."
- Fact: We all need relationships.
- Fact: Belief is more potent than knowledge of the facts.
- Fact: The truth is not the only thing which can set you free.
- Fact: You can only believe in yourself when somebody else has believed in you.
- Fact: You can't give that which you have never received—especially love.
- *New* Fact: we are all capable of offering some kind of help and support.
- *New* Fact: help is closer to you than you think.

~

Probably at several points while reading this book, something inside of you went, "Yes!" You found yourself agreeing with some of the things I have said. I'm not talking about those common-sense ideas that "everybody knows." I am referring to what have been called "A-ha!" moments, when a light-bulb flashes on above your head.

You maybe even had the impression you were learning something new.

Well, no, actually.

As Françoise Dolto has pointed out, when we are able to give our immediate assent to a new idea, then it wasn't new. [18] It struck a chord within us, precisely because we recognised the idea from somewhere else.

However, sometimes it requires particular circumstances in order for such an idea to take shape.

Didier was surprised when I said "Bullshit," but he was not surprised by any new information I had provided. He was simply surprised to hear someone else say it. Hearing it from me enabled him to acknowledge as true what he already suspected. I also enabled him to stop feeling guilty about being unable to see the positive side of things.

Didier recently confided to me that my "Bullshit" that night had made a huge difference in his life. He asked me, "Before you retired, were you a counsellor or a pastor or something like that?"

I gave my own version of the Gallic shrug and said, "The truth is, I read a book once, a long time ago."

If you still feel the need for some kind of official document before allowing others to open up to you, I can provide you with one. First, you will have to take a little exam to prove you have read and understood this book. If you are successful, I will send you a certificate to frame, which will officially testify that... you read a book once.

CHAPTER 11

Is Anybody There?

Flaming red hair and a fiercely bristling red beard. Cold, piercing blue eyes. At least six feet tall. He was a captain of one of those massive oil-tankers. The main reason he had chosen to consult me in particular, was that I lived over a hundred miles from his home and he was unlikely to be seen by anybody he knew.

Overcoming my inclination to say "Yes, sir" every time he opened his mouth, I just listened. He talked about feelings of self-doubt, anxiety, and moments of depression—all "weaknesses" that were unheard of in a merchant navy captain.

At the end, he barked, "So what are you going to do about it?"

"I think you have just done it yourself," I replied.

"What's that supposed to mean?"

"I'm not a gambling man, but I would bet everything I own that this is the first time you have ever spoken to anybody about all that," I told him.

"Of course, it is," he spat out. "You don't think I'm going to let on to any old nincompoop about these shameful, shameful weaknesses. What would they think of me?"

"Well, this nincompoop thinks that you have just committed the greatest act of strength and courage of your life. Well done."

He just looked at me. As I looked back, I noticed tears welling up in his steely blue eyes. A minute later he was weeping like a... Yes, you've got it. Like a baby. He was so physically massive, it seemed as if the whole room trembled as his body was racked with uncontrollable, heaving sobs.

I then said perhaps the most important thing a psychotherapist can say to a patient—nothing. My silent presence was already speaking volumes to him.

When his sobs had died down, I asked, "Would you like a cup of tea before you leave?"

"Is that it?" he queried, with a surprised look.

"What do you think?"

He pulled on his beard and after a moment started nodding his head. "Yes, I think you're right. No milk or sugar, thank you."

I never saw him again, but the next Christmas I received a card from his wife. She just wrote, "I don't know what you did to my husband, but he's a changed man. Thank you, Mr Morgan."

~

When we talk about what is troubling us, there is a therapeutic effect.

We begin to feel better through expressing the thoughts and feelings going on inside of us. Even the language we use to describe this phenomenon is very revealing:

Release.

Open up.

Let it all out.

Get it off my chest.

The implication is there is something which is trying to get out. Something that would actually be better out than in. Khalil Gibran, in *The Prophet*, accurately observed, "You talk when you cease to be at peace with your thoughts." [19] This is always true.

Yet, despite some claims to the contrary, expressing your innermost thoughts to a tree is of very limited usefulness. The act of talking about our issues by itself, is not what brings the therapeutic effect. We talk whenever we want to be heard. To use Gibran's phrasing, we talk about what is troubling us when we hope to attain peace by doing so.

It is commonplace for people to say, "I feel much better now I've been able to talk about all that." It is rarer for people to say the greater truth, "I feel better now that you've listened to me talking about all that." However, this must be the case, otherwise we'd see people talking to trees every time we entered a park.

Therefore, the opening sentence of this section was incomplete.

When we talk to others about what is troubling us, there is a therapeutic effect.

When we talk, we are asking someone to listen to us. The peace we are seeking requires the information we are sharing to be acknowledged. All communication requires not only a sender but a receiver too.

I have asked many people the question, "Why do we communicate?" Very rarely have I received the correct answer. Those who came the closest worked in advertising, for reasons that will become obvious. When communication is taking place, the sender has the intention of modifying the knowledge, attitude, opinions, or behaviour of the receiver. There are no exceptions. Effective communication will accomplish this in the desired way. Flawed communication is the stuff of all human drama.

Maybe you are surprised by my sweeping generalisation. No exceptions? Really?

Yes, really.

Let's take a very simple example. I am walking down the street and I spot somebody I know. I communicate with him by saying, "Hi." At that point I am the sender. In pronouncing that single word, I intend to modify, however briefly, the behaviour of that person. How?

As the sender, I am transmitting the information that:

- I am there.
- I have seen him.
- I am happy to have seen him (communicated by both my tone of voice and my smile).
- I wish him to acknowledge my presence by replying with a greeting or even to stop for a brief chat.

In reacting to my salutation, he in turn, becomes the sender. If he smiles, says "Hi," and stops walking he is informing me that he is happy to see me. He wants me to halt and prolong the exchange. And maybe a dozen other things are going on.

If he looks up, scowls, and walks past me in silence, he is sending another message.

When two sentient beings are aware of each other's presence, communication is happening through words or silences and through their facial expressions and body language. Each one, to a greater or lesser degree, seeks to modify the attitude, opinions, or behaviour of the other.

A helpful regressive relationship is not formed by just unloading our issues on to an unsuspecting family member, friend, or stranger. It is formed when our "Help!" is met by an "OK." When we consult a professional counsellor, we can feel entitled to be listened to, simply because we are paying for that service. Rightly or not, we can feel safe because we have decided to entrust this counsellor with personal information in the hope he will provide us with a solution to our problem. Approaching our family and friends with the same sense of entitlement to be heard and the same expectation of a solution, can be a recipe for disappointment. Not only do we need to be willing to open up, we need to be communicating with someone who is willing to offer help in response to our asking for it.

We all have the potential to be someone's help, but we are all human. Not all of us are willing to be that help... yet.

Your friends and family may not feel able to help you, for they haven't read this book... yet.

Communication is two-way. A sender requires a receiver. A cry for "Help!" needs someone to respond with an "Ok." The baby's cry is reliant upon a mother's care.

Feeling safe.

Feeling heard.

Feeling better.

A therapeutic effect is experienced when we feel cared for in response to asking for help.

So, the opening sentence of this section needs to be modified a final time.

When we talk to others about what is troubling us, there is the therapeutic effect of our being taken care of or feeling cared for.

A need for help meets an offer of help.

A choice to talk meets a choice to listen.

A temporary regressive relationship is created.

And magic happens.

~

There is nothing new is any of this, but....

There's always a "but," isn't there?

But why are we so hesitant to ask for help outside of a therapist's office or a witch-doctor's den? What prevents this exchange from happening in our homes, work places, or communities?

It's not rocket science to ask someone for help, but we refuse to express certain things to others because *we fear their possible reactions*. We believe they will pass judgement on us. Negatively, of course.

Why would we fear negative judgement? Because this would evoke the most basic fear of all humankind. Abandonment. Separation. Rejection. Loss. Alienation. We weren't very happy about it the first time it happened to us when we were ejected from the womb. We don't remember the event, but something remained in us, deeply embedded in some part of our mind, that makes us go to extraordinary lengths to avoid it happening again. Appearances. Conformity. Lies. Half-lies. Lies by omission. Repression. And all the rest.

Why do men, in particular, tend to be so buttoned up? Why did it seem so outrageous for this merchant navy captain to talk about his difficulties?

As we grow up most of us learn to control how we express our feelings and how we react to them. To a large extent, of course, social norms set the limits on what we feel we can express at any given moment. Yet, dismissing the reticence of men to open up as a social phenomenon is an incomplete and unsatisfactory explanation.

I think evolutionary theory has something useful to say about this.

Happiness and comfort are evolutionarily neutral—they do not concern the process of natural selection. However, unhappiness and discomfort are *interpreted* as threats to survival. They therefore provoke avoidance behaviours. It would seem that whether those avoidance behaviours are effective is irrelevant to the survival of the species.

I have tried to find a species where the male can expose his weaknesses with impunity. I couldn't find any. Where male animals are in competition over who gets the girl, they need to show strength not weakness. From shrews to elephants, this demonstration tends to lead to terrifying combat between two males. Male aggression and strength are also required in the competition for territory and resources. It makes no sense, from an evolutionary point of view, for a male to make public the fact that he doesn't "feel up to combat today."

So, from an evolutionary point of view, appearing vulnerable presents more of a threat than an advantage. We are evolutionarily driven to hide our weaknesses.

However, there is an exception to this, for vulnerability characterises a young child.

~

The merchant navy captain drove a hundred miles for what he thought would be some form of clinical hypnosis. Yet, once again, hypnosis played no role. I helped him just by listening. He opened up to me and I failed to judge, despise, or reject him.

I ended up helping him not as "Richard Morgan - Hypnotist" but simply as "Richard Morgan."

The title didn't matter, just my ordinary human presence, albeit within the safety of my office.

Unloading his inner thoughts and feelings brought this captain some relief. But the magic occurred when he broke down and wept. Something happened. I don't know what, and I didn't need to know. Neither did he. Digging for explanations would have been a useless and maybe harmful invasion of his integrity.

I accepted his words and his tears... and then offered him a cuppa. The tea was my way of showing him that I respected what had just taken place.

It has been said (not by me alas), that tears shed in solitude are wasted tears. Tears should be offered to someone. All it takes is for that someone to be there. [20]

“I'm here. I hear you.”

Maybe you could be the someone who is there for somebody who mistakenly believes they have to suffer alone.

CHAPTER 12

How to Listen Effectively

When a person expresses the need to talk about something, the appropriate action to take, if you are feeling so inclined, is to simply be there and listen.

Effective listening is not complicated, but neither is it easy to put into practice.

Firstly, make yourself available so you can be fully present.

A mother responds to her baby's cry for help by putting her own needs on hold. She is not thinking as she hugs her baby, "I wish I could have a moment to talk about my own needs with this kid." She does not say to her child, "Your pain reminds me of a time when I felt something similar..."

To listen effectively, you will need to silence your own needs and issues for as long as the conversation lasts. While somebody is describing to you their anxieties or hurts, you need to ensure you are genuinely mentally available to that person. Nothing else matters. Just like a mother.

An effective gesture can be turning off your mobile phone. Or closing a door. Or moving with them to somewhere quieter.

Your unspoken message must be, "I'm here for you."

Therefore, never offer to listen to someone if you would rather be somewhere else. Do not offer to listen to someone if you haven't got the time to give them your full attention. A person in need of help requires somebody real in front of them, not a charade. In fact, even if you're a great actor/actress, faking being fully present will be sensed. This will prevent the person from being able to open up.

If you have a limited amount of time, just say so. Tell them, "I'd love to talk with you. Let me just say that I will have to go and pick the children up from school at half-past two." Or whatever it is that will pull you away. You could even set a reminder on your phone so you're not worried about checking the time while you listen. You do not need to apologise profusely for having to cut short your time with them. Being straightforward about real commitments in your own life will have the effect of being reassuring. You remove from them any guilt or anxiety they may feel that they are taking up too much of your time. If there is a next time, they will be able to relax into the fact that you are genuinely making yourself available to them, safe in the knowledge that if you have to put an end to the conversation, you will do so, simply and calmly and without reproach.

If you haven't understood something the person has said, be honest about it. "I'm sorry, I didn't understand that. Could you run it by me again, please?" Or if you're struggling to follow the flow of their story, say, "I've heard you say this... have I understood you correctly?" Both interruptions will show you have been listening attentively. The bonus for the person you're listening to, is that repeating something can sometimes be a powerful help. There is a whole school of therapy based around this very principle.

Secondly, accept long silences.

This is not easy. We often become overly self-conscious at times of silence. Our mental availability slips as our own needs begin to demand our attention once again.

Usually, when a person is expressing a problem, lapsing into silence means that something very important is happening inside of them. They have reached a point where they can no longer find the words to express what they are feeling. So, we need to let them have the space to just feel.

If you attempt to get them talking again, in all likelihood you will prevent them from accessing some emotion related to their problem. For most of us, if not all of us, breaking the silence like this is an entirely selfish act. We do it because we feel uncomfortable, not because it is actually helpful to the other person.

You need to be able to allow silence without intruding or interfering. If you should find yourself in this situation, just say to yourself, "There is something happening inside the person opposite me that is infinitely more painful than my discomfort. I will accept feeling ill at ease out of respect for the person who needs my help."

Both your silence and your attention are powerful therapeutic tools.

~

Some people are hesitant to listen to someone in need because they don't know what they would say to them. Why do we imagine that the person opening up needs to have things said to them?

The person sharing with you may well ask questions, such as, "What do you think I should do?" Obviously, this gives the impression that they do want you to say something to them. They may even seem desperate for advice. Don't fall into the trap of answering such questions. A good response is, "Why don't you just carry on sharing with me? I'm no expert, but together we might find something."

Effective listening does not mean giving "good advice." Neither does it mean trying to "fix" or "solve" the other person's problems. You do not need to think of something to say to make the other person feel better. And you certainly do not need to provide any kind of helpful insight into their life. If your focus is upon coming up with these things to say, you will not be fully present with the person sharing.

The things we tend to come out with when we're "thinking of something to say" are often unhelpful to the person sharing. We believe we are making them feel at ease, but we are actually stifling their opportunity to share their pain and problems with us.

Here are some things I recommend you never saying:

"I know exactly how you feel."

You may think this will make the other person feel better. It won't. Because you will have just told them a lie. You have no idea what kinds of emotions are swirling around in the other person's mind, simply because you are not the other person.

"Time heals everything."

This is just another way of saying, "For crying out loud, stop dwelling on it. Just get on with your life and it will pass with time."

"Try to look on the positive side," or *"Count your blessings."*

When did you ever hear this following exchange?

"I've got to go to the dentist. This tooth-ache is excruciating!"

"But you've got no pains in your knees, have you?"

"Dang, you're right. My tooth feels much better now."

Never, that's when.

Sometimes adding up all the positive things that are going on in our lives is not enough to counter the pain that is being experienced.

"I'm sure you'll feel better if you talk things out."

This is another lie. It is highly likely they will feel better, lighter, relieved, and a dozen other pleasant emotions. But you don't know for certain. You can never be sure about the outcome of a person choosing to open up. If the person asks you directly whether talking with you will help them, just remain honest. Tell them, "I don't know. Very often talking something out can make all the difference. I'd certainly be happy to listen, if you feel that's what you want to do." By saying this, you are leaving the person free to hesitate or change their mind half way through.

"Have you tried herbal remedies / going for long walks / asking your doctor for Prozac?"

We think we are helping someone by asking them this kind of question, but by considering the person's possible answers we'll see it is extremely unhelpful. If they haven't tried it, their only answer is, "No." But it implies we think they should stop talking to us and go and try whatever it is, so they can be "fixed." If they have tried it, their only answer is, "Yes, but they didn't help. I still have my problem." Which we already know, because they are still wanting to talk with us about that problem.

~

One of the messages of this book has been that we don't necessarily need to seek out a professional in order to find help. We've all got the potential to help someone in need because we can all listen. We can all respond to a cry for help by offering someone our undivided attention like a mother would to her child.

However, there are times when seeing a professional therapist is essential, for we are rarely in a position to help individuals with serious psychological conditions. People who have a problem with alcohol or drugs will not be helped by a kindly, listening ear. Similarly, people who seriously and frequently threaten to commit suicide or to harm others would need professional help. There are even pathological conditions where the pain of a problem has been present in the person's life for so long that they wouldn't know how to live without it. Paradoxically, they would view moving towards pain-relief as an existential threat.

Most of the people who actually need professional help will seek it out. Most, but not all.

Despite this, that should not prevent us from developing the attitude: I want to be available to listen to those who feel they need to talk. Our willingness to say "Ok" can often help people navigate their way through a storm on the ocean of their life.

Nobody has a one-size-fits-all solution, but sometimes, magic happens.

And now, you know why.

CHAPTER 13

Nothing New Under the Sun

ONEPERSONSINSIGHTCANBEANOTHERPERSONS WHATTHECANTIT

This is how both Ancient Greek and Classical Latin was written. No spaces between words. No punctuation. No uppercase or lowercase distinctions. No clues whatsoever about when one word ended, and another began.

Homer, author of the *Iliad* and the *Odyssey*, wrote like this. The empirical edicts of Julius Caesar were written this way too.

Spaces between words were not introduced into Latin until sometime between 600-800 CE. The modern Greek alphabet—the first to introduce distinct letters for vowels as well as for consonants—was not introduced until somewhere between 700-900 CE.

Text without modern punctuation looks complicated but your familiarity with the English language meant it probably didn't take you too long to add in punctuation, spaces, and lowercase letters:

One person's insight can be another person's, "What the...?" can't it?

Obviously, interpreting the pauses means it took longer to read, but with practise the original audience could make sense of the long, unbroken lines of uppercase Latin or Greek letters ASEASILYASYOUCANMAKESENSEOFTHIS.

However, as we all know, changing the punctuation can totally modify the meaning of a sentence. In spoken English we rely on context and intonation to arrive at the meaning. We have to be a little more careful when we are writing. For example, EATSSHOOTSANDLEAVES could be understood as the eating habits of the koala bear—Eats shoots and leaves—or a brief description of a cold-blooded crime—Eats, shoots, and leaves.

The revelatory experience I was referring to in the jumbled first sentence of the chapter was provoked by a simple comma in the Epistle of James. Since the Christian New Testament was written in Ancient Greek, there were no commas or other punctuation in the original version. How could I be sure that a single comma, so crucial to my flash of insight, had been inserted correctly into the verse in question? After checking all the available Bible translations online in English, French, Portuguese, and Welsh, I was reassured to discover that with only two exceptions, my comma was there.

> Therefore confess your sins to one another, and pray for one another, so that you may be healed. (James 5:16) [21]

The comma I am referring to is the one after the second "another."

To understand my insight, we need to strip away the religious language, which to many of us is irrelevant or even divisive.

Let's replace the word "sins" with "anything we don't want anybody else to know about us." Sharing these things will almost always feel like a "confession." Just as we may feel ashamed of the immoral or unethical things we do, alas we also can feel ashamed of our weaknesses.

When we look at the etymology of the English verb *confess*, we discover that it comes from the Latin *confessare*, a past participle stem of confiteri. "*Con-*" means "together," while "*fiteri*" means "to admit." [22]

Isn't that beautiful?

To admit together.

While "pray for one another," some would argue, has no place in a book about the psychology of human relationships, prayer too has an interesting etymology. We find the root of the English word *pray* is the Latin word *precari*, which means to "ask earnestly, beg, or entreat." [23]

My insight was that the healing the author of James 5:16 talks about could be phrased like this: *To admit together that we need to ask for help from time to time.*

I have not been saying anything different throughout the previous twelve chapters. One could say that my message has been out there for at least two thousand years, perhaps even more.

~

There is a third possibility that sits in between consulting an "expert" and battling on alone in secret.

We can be each other's psychotherapist.

Maybe not all the time. And I am not saying that everybody should share everything with everybody else. Context is everything. But the underlying principles should be the same... in theory.

All the vast varieties of therapy on offer meet with a certain degree of success because they all involve the same essential elements. A demand for help is met by an offer of help. Communication takes place where pain is put into words by one person and is heard by the other.

This doesn't need to occur in an "expert's" office but can happen in a location within our everyday lives where the person sharing feels safe to be heard.

We are all capable of being a good listener. We do this by not judging and by not preaching. Ever. We simply offer our imperfect presence from time to time without expecting a result or a reward. I trust your response to this book will lead to action. Nothing dramatic or world-shattering. Just a small gesture which says, "I'm here. You can be here with me if you want."

And we all need to be the bold sharer occasionally. If at this point in your life, you are in need of help yourself, can I dare you to have the courage to open up to someone you can trust? By doing so, you will be doing a favour to two people, because we all like to be trusted, in case you hadn't noticed. You may also find that being heard is just the remedy you've been looking for.

~

I have a dream. In this dream, somebody who has read this book feels the need to open up about a problem. Instead of making an appointment with a psychiatrist or a marabou, he comes across somebody else who has read this book. This other person has decided he will make himself available to those who need help.

The exchange goes something like this:

"There's something I need to talk about."

"I'm listening."

That's all it takes.

You always knew it. At least you sensed it to be true.

I hope this book will enable you to do it.

ACKNOWLEDGEMENTS

I would like to thank a number of people who have given me their time, precious advice, and helpful criticisms: David Schramm, Frances Janusz, Beth Morgan, Karen O'Dwyer, Aimery Martin, Nicholas Morgan, Graham Robinson, and Christine Biardeau.

—Richard

This collaboration wouldn't have happened without Ian Smith recommending my services. Thanks Ian for introducing Richard to me.

Richard, thank you for trusting me with *Help! OK.* I've enjoyed writing with you immensely, let's do it again in the future.

Carole, your encouragement persuaded me to co-author this book. Thanks for knowing before I did how much I'd enjoy doing it!

—Steve

ABOUT THE AUTHORS

Richard O. Morgan spent ten years as a music teacher before becoming frustrated by his ineffectiveness. He left teaching in 1978 to become a hypnotherapist. As you do. In 1984, he moved from the UK to France, where he became Toulouse's first ever practising hypnotherapist. In 1990 he returned to teaching. Being older and wiser, he fortunately found he was a better teacher. He taught English in the French school system until his retirement in 2011. He continues to live in Toulouse, where he is an official guide at the 13th century church, Notre Dame du Taur.

Steve Hall spent his childhood not knowing what he wanted to do when he became an adult. He enjoyed numbers, so he took a mathematics degree and somehow graduated despite getting more wrong than he got right. Years later, composing essays for a theology degree awakened a dormant love for writing. He was surprised by this too. He is the author of *Lament Forgive* and has now published three books through his business, Cookies and Oxygen Publishing. He and his wife, Carole, have three children and live in South Wales.

If you benefited from reading *Help! OK*, please support Richard and Steve by telling your friends about this book, or by leaving a review in your favourite online bookstore.

ENDNOTES

From CHAPTER 2 *I Wasn't Expecting That*

[1] https://en.oxforddictionaries.com/definition/koan. Accessed September 2018.

[2] Michael Shermer, *Why People Believe Weird Things: Pseudoscience, Superstition, and Other Confusions of Our Time* (Holt Paperbacks, 1997)

From CHAPTER 3 *Jamel and Spinoza*

[3] Baruch Spinoza (Author), Seymour Feldman (Editor), and Samuel Shirley (Translator), *Ethics: Treatise on the Emendation of the Intellect and Selected Letters* (Hackett Classics, [1677] 1992)

[4] Sam Harris, *The Neural Correlates of Religious and Nonreligious Belief* (Annals of Neurology, December 2007)

[5] Robert Burton, *The Certainty Epidemic* (www.salon.com/2008/02/29/certainty/) Accessed September 2018.

[6] William Sargant, *Battle for the Mind: A Physiology of Conversion and Brainwashing* (Heinemann, 1957).

From CHAPTER 5 *What's in a Title?*

[7] Michael Sussman, *A Curious Calling: Unconscious Motivations for Practicing Psychotherapy* (Jason Aronson, 2007)

[8] Robert Epstein Ph.D., and Tim Bower, *Why Shrinks Have Problems* (Psychology Today, July 1997, www.psychologytoday.com/intl/articles/199707/why-shrinks-have-problems) Accessed September 2018.

[9] Robert Epstein Ph.D., and Tim Bower, *Why Shrinks Have Problems* (Psychology Today, July 1997, www.psychologytoday.com/intl/articles/199707/why-shrinks-have-problems) Accessed September 2018.

[10] www.newadvent.org/cathen/01061a.htm. Accessed September 2018.

[11] John Hattie, Christopher F. Sharpley, and H. Jane Rogers, *Comparative Effectiveness of Professional and Paraprofessional Helpers*, (Psychological Bulletin Vol. 95. No. 3, June 1984) 534-541

From CHAPTER 7 *Evolution and Happy Lapses*

[12] R.J. Fitzgibbons Jr. and R.A. Forse, *Clinical Practice. Groin Hernias in Adults* (The New England Journal of Medicine, 372 (8), February 2015) 756–63.

[13] Darwin explained his theory of evolution in his book, *On the Origin of Species* in 1859. He knew nothing about genetics or molecular biology. These recent sciences have led to refinements and modifications of the original theory. For this reason, it is wiser to talk about evolutionary theories in the plural. There is some debate over the causes of genetic mutations, but the process of selection is generally accepted.

From CHAPTER 8 *Placebo/Nocebo. A Science of Care*

[14] Cara Feinberg, *The Placebo Phenomenon: An Ingenious Researcher Finds the Real Ingredients of "Fake" Medicine* (Harvard Magazine, January 2013, https://harvardmagazine.com/2013/01/the-placebo-phenomenon) Accessed September 2018.

[15] Fabrizio Benedetti, Claudia Arduino, and Martina Amanzio, *Somatotopic Activation of Opioid Systems by Target-Directed Expectations of Analgesia* (The Journal of Neuroscience, May 1, 1999, 19(9) 3639–3648, http://www.jneurosci.org/content/19/9/36390). Accessed September 2018.

From CHAPTER 9 *What Actually Happens in Psychotherapy...?*

[16] Dr Nick Read, *Visionary or Disaster; A Perspective on William Sargant* (www.nickread.co.uk/articles/2010/03/visionary-or-disaster-a-perspective-on-william-sargant/) Accessed September 2018.

From CHAPTER 10 *Positively Bullshit*

[17] Françoise Dolto, *Parler juste aux enfants* (Mercure de France, 2002). The English quote is my own translation.

[18] Françoise Dolto, *L'Evangile au risque de la psychanalyse* (France Loisirs, 1978). Published in English as *The Jesus of Psychoanalysis: A Freudian Interpretation of the Gospel* (Doubleday, 1978)

From CHAPTER 11 *Is Anybody There?*

[19] Khalil Gibran, *The Prophet* (1923). The quote is taken from the chapter "On Talking."

[20] I can't remember where I heard those lovely lines about wasted tears. I just know it didn't start with me. I wish it had.

From CHAPTER 13 *Nothing New Under the Sun*

[21] Scripture quotation taken from the New American Standard Bible® (NASB), Copyright © 1960, 1962, 1963, 1968, 1971, 1972, 1973, 1975, 1977, 1995 by The Lockman Foundation. Used by permission. www.Lockman.org

[22] https://www.etymonline.com/word/confess. Accessed September 2018.

[23] https://www.etymonline.com/word/pray. Accessed September 2018.